B

Camel
662091

CASE
STUDIES
IN
PAEDIATRICS

CASE STUDIES IN PAEDIATRICS

David J Field MB, BS(HONS), MRCP(UK), DCH
Research Fellow
Department of Child Health
Nottingham

John Stroobant MB, BS, MRCP(UK), DCH
Research Fellow
Hospital for Sick Children
Great Ormond Street
London

PITMAN

PITMAN BOOKS LIMITED
128 Long Acre, London WC2E 9AN

Associated Companies
Pitman Publishing Pty Ltd, Melbourne
Pitman Publishing New Zealand Ltd, Wellington

First Published 1984

Library of Congress Cataloging in Publication Data
Field, D. (David)
    Case studies in paediatrics.

    1. Pediatrics—Case studies. 2. Pediatrics—Problems,
exercises, etc. I. Stroobant, J. (John) II. Title. [DNLM: 1. Pediatrics—
Problems. WS 18 F453c] RJ58.F54   1984   618.92′009   83-23620
ISBN 0-272-79756-1

British Library Cataloguing in Publication Data
Field, O.
    Case studies in paediatrics.
    1. Paediatrics
    I. Title   II. Stroobant, J.
    618.92   RJ45
    ISBN 0-272-79756-1

Text set in 10/12 pt Linotron 202 Imprint, printed and bound in
Great Britain at The Pitman Press, Bath

The modern MRCP examination demands measurable and high standards of competence while not losing its long-standing status as a difficult examination in elementary medicine. At the level of a postgraduate examination which is to be the entry gate for specialist training, it is therefore necessary that questions should both be crisply worded and contain complex ideas to be sifted and evaluated by the candidate. The collection of questions published in this book, which is based on the realities of clinical practice, will extend and teach the candidate in the course of his preparation for the examination. Many of the questions are difficult and all require careful thought, for none are easy. A few may appear disarming, but none are intended to be deceptive. Each is supplied with appropriate answers and a commentary and the two parts of each teach the candidate a sensible approach to this section of the examination.

It is suggested that the reader, after carefully considering the questions, should first write the answers concisely. It would then be wise to draft some separate paragraphs recording the reader's thoughts and reasoning. Only after this should the candidate refer to the authors' standard answers and commentary. Reviewing this will in turn generate new thoughts and some corrections. At this stage the reader should if necessary consult senior colleagues or reference text to resolve queries and problems and to expand his knowledge. Again, clear notes should be made. The text contains a great deal of material and should be a very useful tool for self instruction which can be annotated as above for revision purposes.

Professor C B S Wood MB, BChir, FRCP, DCH
Academic Department of Child Health
Queen Elizabeth Hospital for Children, London

PREFACE

There is a growing number of books aimed at the candidate taking examinations in Paediatrics. This book developed from a need to have case histories to discuss with candidates as a teaching exercise and is compiled from genuine clinical problems that we have been involved with. Many previously published case histories are artificial and often have a contrived clinical sequence; here, although some details have been pruned and the history has been compressed, we have attempted to put the problem in its genuine clinical setting and have tried to convey the feeling of puzzlement which each of these situations originally gave us. Furthermore, an interest in medical diagnosis should extend beyond preparation for examinations, and we hope that these cases will similarly stimulate an interest in clinical problem solving.

We feel that the cases presented here should be valuable in three areas: as a starting point for discussion with examination candidates (both MRCP(UK) in Paediatrics and DCH), as practice for candidates studying alone; and as a basis for general discussion and approach to clinical problems in any teaching situation.

The answers are not exhaustive, although some discussion is longer where we felt that a fuller explanation was required or where the clinical situation was complicated, requiring a broad investigational approach. There will inevitably be omissions which may partly be explained by differences in approach to any diagnostic problem. The book is not designed to be a discussion of differential diagnosis; however, we give a list of books which we have found useful, both for clinical problems and as an aid to studying for examinations.

Recent Advances in Paediatrics No. 6, Ed. D. Hull. Edinburgh: Churchill Livingstone, 1981.
Textbook of Child Neurology. J. H. Menkes. New York: Lea and Febiger, 1980.
Clinical Paediatric Endocrinology, Ed. C. G. D. Brook. Oxford: Blackwell Scientific Publications, 1981.
Liver Disorders in Childhood. A. P. Mowat. London: Butterworths, 1979.
Textbook of Paediatrics, Ed. J. O. Forfar and G. C. Arneil. Edinburgh: Churchill Livingstone, 1983
Diseases of the Small Intestine in Childhood. J. A. Walker-Smith. London: Pitman, 1979.
Paediatric Chemical Pathology. B. E. Clayton. Oxford: Blackwell Scientific Publications, 1980.
Recognisable Patterns of Human Malformation. D. W. Smith. New York: W. B. Saunders Company, 1982.

We would like to thank Dr Derek Johnston, University Hospital, Queens Medical Centre, Nottingham, for invaluable clinical advice, Katharine Watts, Pitman Books, for her help and encouragement during the preparation of this book, and Mrs Beverley Walker and Mr D A Stainer for their help with the manuscript.

A 4-year-old boy, deeply unconscious, is brought into casualty. He is accompanied only by his grandmother's neighbour. The child's parents have separated and since his mother works he is left during the day with his grandmother who is not very mobile. She was so upset on discovering the boy unconscious that she did not feel able to accompany him to hospital. The neighbour reports that the boy has been really very well, although she thinks his mother has been worried about his gait at some time in the past and he has had a cold during the last few days. After lunch today the boy had gone upstairs to play and grandmother had gone to sleep. She woke at 4.30 p.m. to find the boy on his bed and was unable to arouse him. She therefore dialled 999.

On examination, you find a well nourished boy who is deeply unconscious, not responding to painful stimuli. The boy has wet himself but is not otherwise unkempt. There are bruises on the knees, shins and elbows. His pulse is 40 beats/min, blood pressure 45/20 mmHg but the cardiovascular system is otherwise normal. There is no gag reflex but throat and ears are normal except for blisters on the pinna, and there is another large blister on the back of the hand. The respiratory rate is 10 breaths/min, and there are some crepitations at both lung bases. The reflexes are absent and the child is totally flaccid. Examination of the fundi does not show papilloedema but the veins are dilated.

Sodium	135 mmol/l
Potassium	4.0 mmol/l
Urea	4.0 mmol/l
HCO_3^-	30 mmol/l, $P\text{co}_2$ 7.2 kPa, $P\text{o}_2$ 7.0 kPa (arterial)

Questions

1 What is the diagnosis?
2 What two urgent measures would you undertake?

A 14-month-old Caucasian child is brought into casualty after an illness which has lasted approximately 12 days. The child has had a totally normal neonatal period and childhood up to this point. Twelve days ago he seemed 'unwell' and then parents noticed that his eyes were slightly yellow. The GP visited and diagnosed infectious hepatitis and reassured the parents about the good prognosis. However, during the following few days, the child had remained jaundiced and unwell with vomiting and anorexia. The parents have brought the child up now because, over the last 10 hours, the child has become increasingly 'swollen'. (ascites)

On examination, the child is mildly jaundiced but apyrexial and his general condition is not of urgent concern. There are no signs of chronic liver disease but both legs are grossly oedematous. There is marked ascites and the umbilicus is everted. The spleen is enlarged to 8 cm and a tender liver is palpable 6 cm below the costal margin. There are no other abnormal findings.

Questions

1 What is the most likely diagnosis?
2 How would you confirm this?

A 14-year-old boy presents to his GP having had a right sided convulsion which lasted for 5 minutes. It was his first fit and there was no past history of epilepsy. In his referral letter, the GP reports that the boy has been unwell for about 6 weeks. He was initially seen by a locum who treated an otitis media with penicillin V. Although a perforation occurred, the infection resolved after 5 days of therapy. Having resumed school (4 weeks ago) the boy was rendered unconscious playing rugby and spent a night under observation in the local cottage hospital. During the last 3 weeks the boy has had various complaints, including intermittent pyrexia, unsteady gait and blurred vision.

On examination you find a healthy-looking boy, temperature 38 °C. The left ear drum has a healed perforation with some residual inflammation, but it is not painful. His speech is normal but there appears to be some difficulty in 'subtracting 7s' and he has agnosia for familiar objects. Visual field testing reveals a right homonomous hemianopia. You note some loss of 2 point discrimination but sensation is otherwise normal. There is some weakness on the right side and the right tendon jerk reflexes are brisk. The right plantar reflex is extensor but there is no clonus. The remainder of the examination is normal.

Investigations

Haemoglobin	14.4 g/dl	Sodium	129 mmol/l
White blood count	13×10^9/l	Potassium	3.0 mmol/l
Neutrophils	80%	Urea	2.9 mmol/l
Lymphocytes	19%	HCO_3^-	19 mmol/l
LP cell count – total 150 mm³		Red blood cells	55
		Neutrophils	15
		Lymphocytes	80
		Protein	1 g/l
		Sugar	2.8 mmol/l
		(blood sugar	4.2 mmol/l)

Pressure – not measured

Questions

1 Where is the lesion?
2 What is the most likely diagnosis?
3 What single investigation is the most important?

Answers to case one

1 This boy has taken barbiturates. Points suggesting this are:

  a disrupted social background.
  b general depression of all vital functions.
  c profound neurological disturbance with hypoventilation but without evidence of cerebral irritation or upper motor neurone signs.
  d presence of blisters.
  e hypostatic pneumonia.

2 The following are required:

  a respiratory support.
  b alkaline diuresis.
  c symptomatic treatment as necessary, e.g. plasma infusion for circulatory failure.

An unrelated Caucasian couple have their first child, a boy weighing 3.3 kg, following a 36-hour labour. Membranes had ruptured at onset of labour and oxytocin had been given after 12 hours. Mother had developed a fever of 39°C about 20 minutes before delivery which had been carried out with forceps because of maternal exhaustion. The child's Apgar score at 1 minute was 5 and 9 at 5 minutes. Oxygen was given by mask.

Child and mother went to the ward following an initial normal examination by the obstetrician. During the first 24 hours there were no problems but at 36 hours the midwives noted that the child was lethargic and pale, and was not feeding well. At about 60 hours of life he is found grey and collapsed in his cot. There is now a 3/5 systolic murmur to the left of the pulmonary area, with many crepitations throughout the lung fields. The liver is palpable 2 cm below the costal margin. The bilirubin is 160 μmol/l. Transfer to a neonatal unit is arranged.

Questions

1 What is the most likely diagnosis?
2 What urgent investigation would you undertake?

Answers to case two

1 This boy has acute hepatic vein thrombosis. Points suggesting this are:

a recent jaundice.
b gross hepatosplenomegaly.
c marked peripheral oedema and ascites.
d absence of stigmata of chronic liver disease.

2 Confirmation is by portal venogram and abdominal ultrasound scan.

4 Case Studies in Paediatrics

A 3-year-old girl is taken to her GP because mother thinks she is unwell. She is due to attend a birthday party the next day. The GP diagnoses a viral upper respiratory tract infection, suggests fluids and paracetamol and agrees that the child may attend the party.

The next day the child has a definite cough but is otherwise well and is 'allowed to go to the party. During this, she develops a coughing fit, seems to 'choke' and briefly goes blue. She recovers but has a residual stridor and is taken to casualty. She is examined without any additional physical abnormalities being found and a chest x-ray is normal. The stridor seems to have settled and she is therefore allowed home.

Thirty-six hours later, the child returns with marked stridor and appears cyanosed, temperature 38.5 °C. Her respiratory rate is 60 breaths/min and there is marked intercostal recession. Mother explains that over the last 12 hours the girl has deteriorated rapidly. Further examination reveals her to be very ill with widespread wheezes and crepitations in both lung fields.

Questions

1 What is the diagnosis?
2 What two investigations are required?

Answers to case three

1 *The lesion is in the left temporoparietal area.*
2 *The diagnosis is cerebral abscess. Points suggesting this are:*

   a previous history of infection with inadequate treatment.
   b abnormal physical findings in central nervous system.
   c fever.
   d abnormal CSF finding.
   e slight neutrophilia in blood.

3 *A cerebral CAT scan is the most important investigation. In this situation it is normally wise to delay the lumbar puncture until after the CAT scan has been performed.*

A 14-year-old girl is admitted to hospital with a 2-day history of passing 'smokey' urine which is positive when tested for blood. There was a definite history of an upper respiratory tract infection 2 weeks previously.

Further questioning reveals that she has taken thyroxine from the age of 2 years. At that time, in association with a sore throat, she developed a painful red, midline swelling of the neck which slowly subsided. She later was diagnosed as being hypothyroid.

At the age of 8 years she suffered a further illness with pain in knees, wrists and neck, complicated by heart failure and a rash. She was treated with digoxin, prednisolone and salicylate and, after some weeks' treatment, she was discharged home.

Present investigations		
Sodium	130 mmol/l	
Potassium	4.8 mmol/l	
Urea	6.1 mmol/l	
HCO$_3^-$	18 mmol/l	
Haemoglobin	12.0 g/dl	
White blood count	7.4 × 10⁹/l	(not ↑)
ASOT	400 units/ml ↑	(>100)
BP ↑	140/95 mmHg ↑	

Questions

1 What is the cause of her present illness?
2 What is the cause of the hypothyroidism?
3 What was the illness at 8 years of age?

Answers to case four

✓1 **This baby is in septicaemic shock. Points suggesting this are:**

   a **prolonged rupture of membranes.**
   b **maternal pyrexia.**
   c **clinical status.**
   d **ductus arteriosus opened by septicaemic episode (hypoxia, acidosis).**

2 **An urgent septic screen is required. A primary cardiac lesion must also be considered and investigations would include ECG and echocardiogram.**

A 1-month old baby boy is sent into hospital by his GP with a story that on two occasions he had apparently stopped breathing. Both episodes occurred when the parents were trying to clear the boy's nose with a cotton bud after a feed. The first episode was terminated by stimulation and in the second, the father started mouth to mouth resuscitation. The two events were 7 days apart. The child has an elder brother who has cystic fibrosis but, apart from this, there is no relevant history relating to pregnancy, birth or family illness.

On examination in hospital, he is well nourished and not distressed. He is pink in air. Several initial investigations are performed, including an urgent sweat test and it is planned to carry out a period of observation. Eighteen hours later, an arrest call is put out and the arrest team arrives to find a white, shocked baby with gasping respirations. The nurse in charge reports that the child had been very distressed without his mother and had been crying incessantly for about 4 hours prior to this spontaneous respiratory arrest.

Investigations

Haemoglobin	14.1 g/dl
White cell count	15.0×10^9/l
Neutrophils	65%
Lymphocytes	31%
Monocytes	2%
Eosinophils	2%
Sodium	132 mmol/l
Potassium	4.1 mmol/l
Urea	4.0 mmol/l
HCO_3^-	25 mmol/l
Sweat test	Sodium 55 mmol/l, weight of sweat 85 mg
Stool microscopy	No fat globules seen
Chest x-ray	Some overinflation

Question

What is the diagnosis?

Answers to case five

1 *This little girl had inhaled a peanut at the birthday party. Points suggesting this are:*

  a *history of choking attack.*
  b *deterioration over 36 hours.*
  c *widespread pulmonary signs.*

  Viral croup and epiglottitis are important in the differential diagnosis.

2 *Bronchoscopy is urgently required and x-ray of chest and airways help in distinguishing an infectious aetiology.*

A 7-year-old boy is referred for admission by his GP because, during the course of a febrile illness with rash, he has become jaundiced. The boy had been perfectly well until 6 days previously when he developed a fever and malaise, which lasted for 48 hours before he developed a macular rash. The fever and malaise continued for another 4 days before he started passing red-brown urine and 24 hours later was first noted to be jaundiced. He had also developed a diffuse myalgia.

On examination, he is well grown with yellow sclerae and has a liver palpable 1 cm below the costal margin; the spleen is not palpable.

He is one of four children, all of whom had been well, except for his elder brother, now aged 13, who had had severe jaundice in the neonatal period. This had been investigated and treated in Greece where the family were living at the time. Mother is 41 years of age, of Greek origin, and has thalassaemia minor. Father is 47 years of age and well. He was originally an export salesman who had taken up farming 5 years previously. The family now live on a dairy farm.

Investigations

Haemoglobin	10.1 g/dl
White blood count	8.2×10^9/l
Platelets	300×10^9/l (>150K) -(ot-penia)
Sodium	141 mmol/l
Potassium	3.9 mmol/l
Urea	4.1 mmol/l
HCO_3^-	24 mmol/l
Bilirubin	32 μmol/l
Urinalysis	Blood +, Urobilinogen + +, Bilirubin 0
Abdominal ultrasound scan	Within normal limits

Questions

1 Give the most likely diagnosis.
2 How would you confirm the diagnosis?
3 What is the prognosis?

Answers to case six

1 The girl currently has post-streptococcal glomerulonephritis. Points suggesting this are:

a previous history of throat infection.
b passing smokey urine.

2 Her hypothyroidism was the result of an acute infective thyroiditis.
3 At 8 years of age she developed juvenile chronic polyarthritis. The presence of cervical arthritis makes this diagnosis more likely than rheumatic fever.

A boy aged 18 months presents to the outpatients department. The parents explain that the child has had a problem with rapid breathing since birth. Although never cyanosed, he was fully investigated, including cardiac catheterization at the age of 10 days, with no abnormal findings. Since that time he has had two episodes of pneumonia requiring hospital admission but these had responded promptly to antibiotics.

His perinatal history, other than the tachypnoea, had been unremarkable; birth weight 3.4 kg. He was successfully breast fed for 5 months.

On examination, his height and weight are below the third centile while his head circumference is on the third centile. He has a respiratory rate of 50 breaths/min and an immobile small chest is noted. There are no added sounds on auscultation. The remainder of the examination is normal.

Investigations

Haemoglobin	13.2 g/dl
White blood count	6.0×10^9/l
Normal differential	
Sodium	135 mmol/l
Potassium	4.1 mmol/l
Urea	3.2 mmol/l
Creatinine	16 mmol/l

pH 7.33, P_{O_2} 11.5 kPa, P_{CO_2} 6.5 kPa,
Standard HCO_3^- 27 mmol/l, standard base excess +3.1 mmol/l

Questions

1 What is the diagnosis?
2 How would you confirm the diagnosis?
3 What is the prognosis?

Answers to case seven

This child died 4 weeks later from cystic fibrosis having marked lung disease which was clinically not apparent, despite the chest x-ray findings. The family history obviously points to this diagnosis. The sweat test was invalid because of an inadequate weight of sweat.

A girl of 6 months is brought to the casualty department totally unresponsive. Mother reports that the child had been mildly unwell for 36 hours and today was unable to rouse the child from her afternoon nap. Previously, the child had been well, apart from a tendency to bruise easily. Mother had discussed this fully with the clinic doctor who had reassured her that the bruises were of no consequence. The child's perinatal history had been uneventful.

There are no other children in the family and no history of disease in close relatives. Father, aged 28, is unemployed, and mother, aged 26, now a housewife, had previously worked in a children's home. She had been an orphan from the age of 6 years.

The child is acutely ill and retinal haemorrhages are noted, with bilateral VI nerve palsies. There are bruises on her chest and legs but no obvious signs of injury to the head.

Questions

1 What is the diagnosis?
2 What would be one test to confirm the diagnosis?

Answers to case eight

1 *This boy has glucose-6-phosphate dehydrogenase deficiency. This attack has been triggered by an intercurrent infection. Points suggesting this diagnosis are:*

   a *Greek mother (sex-linked recessive disorder).*
   b *brother's history.*
   c *onset of jaundice following infection.*
   d *mild jaundice with increased urobilinogen in the urine.*
   e *haemoglobinuria.*
   f *mild anaemia.*

2 *Confirmation of the diagnosis involves measurement of red cell enzyme level.*
3 *Prognosis is excellent.*

You are called to see a 12-hour-old baby boy, weighing 4.1 kg. His delivery was normal at term. Mother had been well during pregnancy apart from some minimal intermittent glycosuria. Father is a severe epileptic and works for the Forestry Commission.

The midwives had noticed increasing tachypnoea over the previous 2–3 hours and the child now appears dusky. The baby is otherwise well and 2 hours previously had taken his feed without difficulty.

On examination, the child is tachypnoeic, 80 breaths/min, and mildly cyanosed. The cardiovascular system appears normal. However, examination of the chest reveals absent breath sounds over the left upper zone. The abdomen and central nervous system are normal.

The child is placed in an incubator with 35% O_2, and although he readily becomes pink, the dyspnoea does not settle. A chest x-ray reveals a cavity in the upper half of the left hemithorax and within this, a clear fluid level of approximately 3 cm diameter.

Questions

1 Give two possible diagnoses.
2. Give two useful investigations.
3 What is the treatment for your first diagnosis?

Answers to case nine

1 This boy has asphyxiating thoracic dystrophy of Jeune. Points suggesting this are:

a persistent tachypnoea without lung parenchymal or cardiovascular cause.
b small stature.
c chest deformity.
d mild chronic respiratory acidosis.

2 Diagnosis is confirmed by x-rays of ribs (short and hypoplastic) and pelvis (broad) which have a characteristic appearance.

3 Prognosis is variable, but is good after the first year of life providing that respiratory failure does not supervene. Renal failure, because of the association of dysplastic kidneys, may complicate the course.

A 4-year-old boy is brought to the casualty department lethargic and hypoventilating. Within a few minutes of arrival he has a respiratory arrest and requires intubation. He responds quite rapidly to bagging and is extubated 7 minutes later. He manages to maintain his respiration for approximately 15 minutes when he has a further respiratory arrest. He is reintubated and ventilated.

History from the parents reveals that the boy has been unwell intermittently over the preceding 2 weeks, initially with a cold and cough, and subsequently with lethargy and inactivity, but without specific symptoms.

On examination, while being ventilated, he appears rather hypotonic and reflexes are difficult to elicit. His face is expressionless. You note that his knees are badly bruised and mother explains he has had one or two nasty tumbles in the preceding 2 days.

Investigations

Haemoglobin	14.3 g/dl
White cell count	7.1×10^9/l
Differential is normal	
Sodium	142 mmol/l
Potassium	4.1 mmol/l
Urea	6.1 mmol/l
HCO_3^-	29 mmol/l
Glucose (random)	5.0 mmol/l

Questions

1 What is the most likely diagnosis?
2 How would you confirm the diagnosis?
3 What is the long term prognosis?

Answers to case ten

1 *This girl in fact had haemophilia A and has suffered an intracranial haemorrhage. Non-accidental injury, of course, needs consideration. Von Willebrand's disease is also possible from the history. Points suggesting this are:*

a previous history of bruising.
b lack of signs of trauma to explain this present episode.

2 *Confirmation is by clotting studies, factor VIII assay, and platelet function studies.*

A 7-year-old boy is referred to hospital by his GP. The boy had been perfectly well until a year previously when he developed a crowing stridor, following a mild upper respiratory tract infection. In every other way he was well. He is the elder child in the family, having a younger brother aged 4 months. His parents are both 23 years of age and well, but of quite limited intelligence. Four years previously the social services department had been involved with this family, investigating allegations of child abuse, but the contact had lapsed during the social workers' strike. Much of the impetus for this present referral has come from the boy's school who found the stridor very distracting in the classroom.

On examination, the boy demonstrates a marked inspiratory stridor of crowing quality, but this is very variable and when quiet and not agitated the boy is able to breathe noiselessly. The rest of the examination is normal, the tonsils are not large and the voice is apparently normal. At night asleep, the stridor becomes gross and there are episodes of near respiratory obstruction.

Investigations

Chest x-ray	Normal
Barium swallow	Normal
Lateral x-ray of chest/ head/neck	Moderate adenoidal pad.
Blood gases	pH 7.32, P_{CO_2} 7 kPa, P_{O_2} 10 kPa, HCO_3^- 27 mmol/l
Laryngoscopy and bronchoscopy under general anaesthetic	Normal findings
Serum calcium	Normal

Questions

1 What two diagnoses would you consider?
2 Give two further investigations.
3 What therapeutic measure is likely to be required?

Answers to case eleven

1 *This child has a cystic adenomatous malformation of the upper lobe of the left lung, although on the evidence given it is not possible to differentiate this from a diaphragmatic hernia.*
Significant points are:

   a *early onset of respiratory distress.*
   b *response of cyanosis to oxygen.*
   c *chest x-ray signs.*

2 *Useful investigations for making a specific diagnosis include:*

   a *plain abdominal x-rays and lateral chest x-ray (looking for bowel gas pattern and clear diaphragmatic outlines).*
   b *abdominal x-ray with nasogastric tube in place.*
   c *Gastrografin swallow.*

3 *Treatment is surgical for both conditions.*

A 10-month-old female infant is sent into hospital by the GP because over the preceding 3 weeks there have been increasing difficulties with feeds. The child had been born at home, a normal delivery at term. There had been no problems until about $8\frac{1}{2}$ months of age when she had a severe upper respiratory tract infection. She recovered over 7 days and had been well for about 1 week when the feeding problems commenced. Initially, the child was a little more miserable than previously and at times tended to 'fight' when being fed. Over the week prior to being admitted she had been vomiting increasing amounts of her feeds.

Her mother is 26 and well. Father is 27 and suffers from ankylosing spondylitis. He has HLA B_{27} and family studies have already revealed that the little girl also has HLA B_{27}. Her brother is HLA B_{27} negative and quite well.

On examination, the child appears slightly dehydrated and tachypnoeic, 45–50 breaths/min, but otherwise there are no abnormal findings.

Investigations

Haemoglobin	14.1 g/dl
White cell count	6.4×10^9/l
ESR	7 mm/h
Sodium	130 mmol/l
Potassium	3.9 mmol/l
Urea	7.8 mmol/l
HCO_3^-	16 mmol/l
pH	7.32
P_{CO_2}	3.2 kPa
P_{O_2}	10.1 kPa
Chest x-ray	Normal

Questions

1 What is the most likely diagnosis?
2 Give the three most important subsequent investigations.

Answers to case twelve

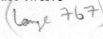

(Lange 767)

1 This boy has the Guillain–Barré syndrome. Points suggesting this are:

a onset following infection.
b evidence of recent weakness, now increased and involving the muscles of respiration.
c facial palsy.
d lower motor neurone signs.

2 Diagnosis is best confirmed by lumbar puncture to demonstrate raised CSF protein without increase in cells.

3 Generally, the long term outlook for recovery is good. Controlled trials show that there is no routine place for corticosteroids. Plasmaphaeresis may help in chronic cases.

A male infant returns to outpatients at the age of 12 weeks with failure to thrive. He was born at 39 weeks, a normal delivery, birth weight 3.7 kg. He was breast fed and discharged at 48 hours, well, apart from some mild snuffles.

At home mother found that the snuffling became worse and he developed a mild cough. When weighed, aged 3 weeks, at his local child health clinic, he had lost 200 g and he was admitted to hospital for observation of his feeding pattern. It was decided that his mother's supply of breast milk was inadequate and his feeds were changed to 'humanized' cows' milk, 160 ml/kg.

On this regimen the child gained 200 g over the next 3 weeks but was more chesty. Following a diagnosis of cows' milk allergy, his feeds were changed to a soya based formula. Over the next 6 weeks his symptoms of coughing and poor weight gain continued and when attending outpatients at 12 weeks, mother comments that recently he has had a tendency to wheeze and has developed small pustules on his face and arms.

Questions

1 What is the diagnosis?
2 Give two tests to confirm this.

Answers to case thirteen

1 This boy has bilateral vocal cord palsy, although in view of the essentially normal examination a psychological basis for his symptoms was considered. Points in favour of the former are:

a presence of stridor during sleep.
b evidence of CO_2 retention.
c all common causes excluded by investigations already performed.

Diagnosis is made by assessing vocal cord movement, during recovery from anaesthesia. A normal range of movement should occur.

2 Investigations to consider looking for a possible underlying pathology are:

a cerebral CAT scan.
b nerve conduction studies.

3 Treatment, if airway is compromised, is by tracheostomy until growth of the larynx is complete.

A male infant of 8 weeks is brought to casualty at 4 a.m. by his parents. He has been unwell with a cough and fever for 3 days and has been receiving amoxycillin from the GP. Over the last 12 hours his general condition worsened and now he is extremely ill.

He is the second child of unrelated parents. Their first child, a boy, had died aged 5 weeks with *Pneumocystis carinii* pneumonia. Both parents are young and healthy with no history of familial illness.

This child was a normal delivery at term, birth weight 3.7 kg and was bottle fed from birth. He had smiled at 4 weeks and his parents were very satisfied with his progress until this recent episode.

On examination, he appears pale and listless, with an unrecordable blood pressure. At this point he stops breathing and requires intubation. This is made difficult by the presence of fresh blood in the trachea. Once mechanical ventilation is established the rest of the examination is completed and reveals marked bruising but no other significant abnormalities, although at this stage the child is unconscious.

Clotting studies show disseminated intravascular coagulation.

Questions

1 What is the diagnosis?
2 What underlying pathology should you consider?

Answers to case fourteen

1 This child has diabetes mellitus. Points suggesting this are:

  a increasing misery.
  b vomiting.
  c dehydration.
  d metabolic acidosis.

  Other causes of metabolic acidosis also need to be excluded and infection, e.g. urinary tract, considered.

2 Useful investigations include:

  a blood sugar.
  b routine urine test for sugar, ketones and pH.
  c urine culture.
  d blood culture.
  e urinary amino and organic acids.
  f serum lactate and pyruvate.
  g LP

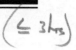

A 4-year-old boy is seen in outpatients with a history of several months' irritability and 'tetchiness' in the mornings. He always seems better after breakfast. On four occasions he has apparently blacked out, collapsed onto the floor and twitched for a few minutes.

He had been delivered with the aid of forceps at 39 weeks for delay in the second stage. Apgar scores had been normal and no resuscitation was required. Birth weight was 2.4 kg. There had been no subsequent problems and for 2 years he was followed in the hospital baby clinic during which time he grew parallel to, but below, the 3rd centile. His present weight is consistent with that trend. His height is on the 20th centile.

On examination, he appears to have normal development for a 4-year-old and the only positive finding is a liver edge palpable 2 cm below the costal margin. The spleen is not palpable.

Investigations

Haemoglobin	14.1 g/dl
White cell count	7.3×10^9/l
Normal differential	
Sodium	132 mmol/l
Potassium	4.5 mmol/l
Urea	6.1 mmol/l
HCO_3^-	23 mmol/l
Calcium	2.31 mmol/l
PO_4	1.1 mmol/l
Alkaline phosphatase	541 U/l
Bone age at wrist	3 years

Questions

1 What is the most likely cause for the presenting problem?
2 Give two tests to confirm your answer.

Answers to case fifteen

1 This child has cystic fibrosis. Points suggesting this are:

   a failure to thrive despite adequate intake.
   b persistent chest signs.

2 Confirmation can be by:

   a sweat test.
   b duodenal intubation and analysis of pancreatic secretion.
   c immunotrypsin assay. May be unreliable at this age.

A 10-week-old female infant is referred to hospital by the local infant welfare clinic because of persistent jaundice. The child was a normal delivery at term and had been discharged, breast fed, at 48 hours. She was first noted to be jaundiced by the midwife at day 5, along with a fading petechial rash, but neither seemed severe. However, the jaundice had not decreased by the next regular review at the clinic and, although the doctor there had initially felt quite confident that this was simply a breast milk jaundice, the poor weight gain from 2.8 kg at birth to 4.1 kg now made him feel that further examination and investigation was required.

Her parents are both 24 years of age. Father is a pharmacist and suffers from diabetes mellitus. Mother, an ex-nurse, is well, although she did have a 'flu-like' illness during the third trimester of this pregnancy. There is a 4-year-old sister who is normal.

On examination, you find a small infant with definite jaundice but no signs of chronic liver disease. Examination of the cardiovascular, respiratory and central nervous systems is normal. Examination of the abdomen reveals a firm liver edge, palpable 4 cm below the costal margin and a spleen palpable 3 cm below the costal margin. The stools are very pale.

Investigations

Sodium	130 mmol/l
Potassium	4.1 mmol/l
Urea	5.1 mmol/l
HCO_3^-	21 mmol/l
AST	104 U/l
ALT	94 U/l
Haemoglobin	9.9 g/dl
White blood count	7.2×10^9/l
Urine testing	Bilirubin +
^{131}I Rose Bengal excretion at 72 hours	10%
Bilirubin	222 μmol/l (conjugated 200 μmol/l, unconjugated 22 μmol/l)

Questions

1 What is the diagnosis?
2 Give six useful investigations.
3 What do you suggest is the underlying pathology here?

Answers to case sixteen

1 **Septicaemia.**

2 *This child was immunocompromised and in fact had severe combined immune deficiency. Points suggesting this are:*

a *rapid progression of infective signs in a previously well child.*
b *past history of sibling dying of pneumocystis pneumonia.*

A 3-month-old female infant is readmitted from the outpatient department. The follow-up had been arranged originally because during the neonatal period, the child had developed intestinal obstruction and at laparotomy had bowel resected for what appeared to be Hirschsprung's disease. This was confirmed on histological examination.

Following discharge, the parents had increasing difficulty in getting the child to take feeds. At the same time the child had become constipated. The parents also feel that the little girl is not as alert and active as their other child had been at the same age. Mother is 28 and well and father 41, a bank manager, is also well.

On examination, the child is rather floppy and there is an umbilical hernia. She sits with her tongue protruding as if the mouth were too small to fit it in, and she is rather snuffly. The neck appears short with supraclavicular fat pads and her hair is thin.

Questions

1 What is the diagnosis?
2 How is this most easily confirmed?
3 What is the prognosis?

Answers to case seventeen

1 This child is having hypoglycaemic fits secondary to ketotic hypoglycaemia. Points suggesting this are:

a small-for-dates infant.
b relatively underweight for height. (lean)
c fits occur after overnight fast.
d age of onset.

However, the following conditions also need consideration.

a glycogen storage disease.
b growth hormone deficiency.
c hypothyroidism.
d adrenal insufficiency.

2 Useful investigations include:

a monitored fast with serial blood sugar measurement. Hypoglycaemia with keto-nuria suggests a substrate deficiency, an enzyme block or endocrine deficiency. Hypoglycaemia without ketonuria suggests hyperinsulinism. Measurement of growth hormone, cortisol, insulin, lactate and ketone bodies during spontaneous hypoglycaemia usually avoids the need for other provocative studies.
b blood sugar and lactate response to intramuscular glucagon.
c growth hormone level during fasting.

A 7-year-old girl is sent by her GP because of symptoms of increasing cough and breathlessness for 4 weeks, despite a course of co-trimoxazole and later ampicillin. The GP feels there are signs of pulmonary consolidation which are not resolving.

Mother explains that the whole family (father and her brothers, aged 4 and 9) have had some form of virus and even the guinea pig has seemed unwell. Everyone else, however, recovered after a few days. Father's health has not been good for some years and he attends his GP regularly with chronic fibrositis.

On examination, the child is apyrexial but does not look entirely well with a respiratory rate of 40 breaths/min. Expansion of the left chest is limited with some dullness to percussion over a similar area. Breath sounds at the left base are considerably reduced but are bronchial in the mid zone. The admission weight shows the girl to have lost 3 kg in the last month.

Investigations

Haemoglobin	9.8 g/dl	Mantoux 1 in 1000	Negative
Reticulocytes	9%	Sodium	138 mmol/l
WBC	16×10^9/l	Potassium	4.1 mmol/l
Neutrophils	78%	Urea	4.1 mmol/l
Lymphocytes	20%	HCO_3^-	23 mmol/l

Questions

1 What is the most likely diagnosis?
2 Give two tests to confirm this.
3 What is the appropriate treatment?

Answers to case eighteen

1 This child has the neonatal hepatitis syndrome although it is not possible to exclude biliary atresia. Points in favour of either diagnosis are:

a prolonged jaundice.
b poor weight gain.
c pale stools.
d hepatosplenomegaly.
e abnormal liver function tests.

Points in favour of the neonatal hepatitis syndrome are:

a petechiae present at the time of birth.
b history of flu-like illness in last trimester.

The Rose Bengal excretion result is equivocal.

2 Investigations:

a congenital infection screen.
b plasma and urine amino acids.
c alpha-1 antitrypsin phenotype.
d sweat test.
e urine reducing substances.
f urine culture.
g ultrasound scan of abdomen.
h thyroid function (typically unconjugated jaundice in hypothyroidism).
i liver biopsy.

3 The baby had congenital cytomegalovirus infection although the history of a flu-like infection in the last trimester and petechiae in the first week of life would also be compatible with toxoplasmosis infection.

A male infant, aged 54 hours, is transferred to the special care baby unit from the postnatal ward because of increasing lethargy and poor feeding. During the last 2–3 hours the baby had at times seemed jittery and just before leaving the postnatal ward, had had a generalized convulsion.

The baby was delivered by Kjelland's forceps because of occipito posterior position. Apgar scores were 5 at 1 minute, 8 at 5 minutes and 10 at 10 minutes. Birth weight was 3.8 kg. No active resuscitation had been required.

This pregnancy had been quite uneventful. Mother, a 23-year-old Cypriot housewife, was well but had lost a full term baby in Cyprus. At a few days of age it had become comatose and had subsequently died at 10 days. The parents had been told that this first child, also a boy, had died as a result of a 'brain condition'. The father, a 37-year-old restaurant owner, and also the mother's first cousin, was very well. The only illness he had suffered was gonorrhoea when aged 21. They had come to England 2½ years previously.

consanguinity

On examination, the child is generally rather hypertonic and inactive but very irritable when disturbed. The rest of the examination is normal and he passes urine with a good stream during the examination. An hour after the initial move to the special care baby unit, he develops apnoea and artificial ventilation is started.

Investigations

Haemoglobin	14.1 g/dl
White blood count	8.3×10^9/l
Sodium	139 mmol/l
Potassium	4.1 mmol/l
Urea	4.1 mmol/l
LP	1 rbc/mm³, 1 wbc/mm³ *(NORMAL)*
	No organisms
Chest x-ray	Normal
Skull x-ray	Normal

Questions

1 What is the likeliest diagnosis?
2 Give three important investigations.
3 Give three general therapeutic measures to be undertaken.

Answers to case nineteen

1 This child has Down's syndrome. Points suggesting this are:

a presence of Hirschsprung's disease.
b poor feeding.
c hypotonia.
d tongue protruding from small mouth.
e snuffly.
f short neck with supraclavicular fat pads.

Some of this description would also be compatible with a child with hypothyroidism.

2 Diagnosis is confirmed by chromosome analysis.

3 Prognosis is for a child in the ESN (S) range of intellect.

A 5-day-old baby is admitted to the children's ward at the request of the health visitor, who has been very worried about the baby since discharge from hospital at 48 hours. The baby was the second child of healthy young parents whose eldest child, now aged 4 years, is quite well. The child was grossly floppy with no spontaneous movement of his limbs although he had minor twitches of the fingers which seemed to occur intermittently. However, he was taking his feeds well and seemed alert and interested in his surroundings. He cried little and never very loudly.

The child had been delivered by his GP in hospital who had not examined the baby before discharge as he had intended to do this at home at the end of the first week. Examination now confirms the above physical abnormalities and provides the additional information that the tendon and plantar reflexes are absent.

Investigations

Haemoglobin	18.4 g/dl
White cell count	12.1×10^9/l
Sodium	136 mmol/l
Potassium	4.5 mmol/l
Urea	4.3 mmol/l
HCO_3^-	26 mmol/l
Bilirubin	162 μmol/l
AST	16 U/l
ALT	14 U/l
Alkaline phosphatase	79 U/l (56–160)
CPK	100 U/l (8–60 U/l)

Questions

1 What is the diagnosis?
2 How would you confirm this?

Answers to case twenty

1 This little girl has Mycoplasma pneumoniae *pneumonia. Points suggesting this are:*

　a *chest symptoms and signs of consolidation.*
　b *weight loss.*
　c *failure to respond to ampicillin and co-trimoxazole.*
　d *haemolytic anaemia.*

2 Confirmation of the diagnosis can be by:

　a *growing the organism.*
　b *rise in antibody titres to* Mycoplasma pneumoniae.
　c *presence of cold agglutinins.*
　d *presence of antibodies to streptococcus M G.*

3 Treatment of choice is erythromycin.

A 6-month-old infant is admitted as an emergency with an acutely inflamed left foot. He had been born at 30 weeks' gestation and was an inpatient for 8 weeks. Since then he had been very well and had 3 days earlier attended hospital for a full blood count as part of his prematurity follow-up. Over the 24 hours prior to admission the child had seemed hot and miserable and not interested in feeds. The parents took him to the GP's surgery who felt admission was indicated.

Examination reveals an acutely inflamed, swollen left foot, maximum swelling being centralized around the ankle.

Questions

1 Give the most likely diagnosis.
2 Give three useful investigations.

Answers to case twenty-one

1 The boy has an inborn error of metabolism involving the urea cycle. Points suggesting this are:

a fitting and cerebral irritation but with no evidence of central nervous system infection.
b loss of previous child.
c parents first cousins.
d timing of onset of problems.
e absence of metabolic acidosis.

(atypical compared to other) metabolic effects

Septicaemia should be considered.

2 Investigations could include:

a serum ammonia.
b serum lactate and pyruvate.
c serum and urine amino acids.
d blood gas analysis.

3 Treatment involves:

a intravenous infusion of dextrose and electrolytes until clinical status stabilizes (bicarbonate dialysis often needed).
b cautious reintroduction of restricted protein, possibly adding keto acids.

A 7-year-old West Indian boy presents to casualty with a 12-hour history of abdominal pain. The pain is fairly constant and centred around the umbilicus. He has felt sick almost from the onset, has vomited twice but has eaten nothing and drunk only sips. He has not had his bowels open for 24 hours, the last stool being normal. The boy's mother has been rubbing his abdomen with warm oil and this seems to be helpful in relieving the pain. Mother is particularly worried since the boy normally drinks so much and is now refusing fluids.

The boy is one of four children, the others, all boys, are 13, 11 and 4 years. The mother is unmarried and the family live in a delapidated council house next to a factory which makes car batteries.

Examination reveals a tall, thin boy with diffuse tenderness of the lower abdomen. His temperature is 38°C. Apart from a slightly inflamed throat there are no abnormal findings.

Investigations

Haemoglobin	8.0 g/dl
White cell count	13.6 × 10⁹/l
Neutrophils	80%
Lymphocytes	19%
Sodium	139 mmol/l
Potassium	4.4 mmol/l
Urea	3.1 mmol/l
HCO_3^-	18 mmol/l
Abdominal x-ray	Normal
Chest x-ray	Normal

Questions

1 Give the three most likely diagnoses.
2 Give three useful investigations.

Answers to case twenty-two

1 This child has Werdnig–Hoffmann disease. Points suggesting this disorder are:

a early onset of weakness.
b gross hypotonia.
c absence of movement.
d fasciculation of fingers.
e absent tendon jerk reflexes.

2 Investigations should exclude other possible causes such as congenital myopathy, myasthenia or a cervical cord lesion.

a nerve and muscle conduction studies.
b muscle biopsy.
c cervical spine x-ray.
d 'Tensilon' test.

A 17-month-old female infant is referred because of delayed walking. The child had a normal delivery at term. During the pregnancy the mother had severe problems with morning sickness but once this settled she had been well. The baby was breast fed, there had been no neonatal problems, and she was well on discharge. At the age of 6 weeks, the mother had felt that the infant was not satisfied and changed the feeds to 'humanized' milk which caused the infant to become constipated. The health visitor suggested adding brown sugar and water and this relieved the problem. Smiling commenced around the sixth week. At this time the child was showing definite responses to sounds and bright objects. By 7 months, the child was able to sit and show interest in objects with which she would play for minutes at a time. By 10 months, the child was quite mobile and could shuffle around quite freely on her bottom. By one year, she could say two or three words but understood several more. Now, at 17 months, she knows many more words but can still only bottom shuffle. Over the past one or two weeks she seemed to be trying to pull to stand. She is wet night and day and feeds herself only with difficulty. She seems to dislike being dressed and does not cooperate in any way. She is not hypotonic.

Her parents are naturally anxious since this is their first child. Mother is 26 and well. Father is a 45-year-old accountant who is well and who ran for Cambridge as a student. He is keen that everything possible should be done for the child.

Questions

1 What do you consider is the pathology here?
2 What is the prognosis for walking?

Answers to case twenty-three

1 This child has osteomyelitis following the heel prick made when attending for repeat full blood count. Points suggesting this are:

a history of heel prick.
b physical findings in foot.

2 Investigations could include:

a blood culture.
b needle aspiration.
c x-rays of foot for later comparison (acute osteomyelitis would not show bone changes at this stage).
d bone scan.
e investigation of immune system.

A 34-year-old Maltese woman in her sixth pregnancy is admitted at 34 weeks in strong labour, membranes having ruptured at home some 4 hours earlier. She progresses to a breech delivery of a male infant weighing 1.9 kg. Apgar score at 1 minute is 1 and the child at that point is intubated and given intermittent positive pressure ventilation. There follows an initial improvement in heart rate but no change in colour and the heart rate soon deteriorates again. At 7 minutes it appears that the child has bilateral pneumothoraces with minimal air entry on both sides. Two chest drains are inserted but no improvement occurs, although some air is evacuated and a slight swing is noted in the drains. Despite further resuscitative manoeuvres the child dies at 35 minutes of age.

After death, the only additional abnormalities noted are low set ears, and there appears to be an excessive amount of skin, particularly over the limbs where there are extra skin folds.

Questions

1 At 7 minutes of life, give three important points of management not mentioned.
2 What is the likely pathology here?

Answers to case twenty-four

1 *This boy was in fact suffering a sickle cell pain crisis. Points suggesting this are:*

a *West Indian origin.*
b *polydipsia.*
c *mild fever.*
d *anaemia.*

However, the differential diagnosis includes the following:

a *diabetes mellitus.*
b *lead poisoning.*
c *mesenteric adenitis.*
d *urinary tract infection.*
e *appendicitis.*

2 *With these possibilities in mind, useful investigations would be:*

a *sickle screen and haemoglobin electrophoresis.*
b *blood glucose.*
c *blood lead level.*
d *urine examination and culture.*
e *rectal examination.*
f *stool for bacteriology/virology.*

A 7-year-old girl is referred by her school doctor because of a deterioration in her school performance in the previous 6–9 months. Up to that time she had been a bright, lively little girl but lately had become rather uninterested in school.

On examination, she looks well. Her pulse rate is 55 beats/min but otherwise the cardiovascular system is normal. The only other abnormal finding is an anterior swelling in the neck. The mother reports that this had been present from about 18 months of age and has slowly been getting bigger.

The child has another sister, aged 3 years, who has a similar swelling. Mother and father are both young and fit. The maternal grandmother and a maternal aunt take thyroxine for myxoedema, presenting in the fourth and third decades respectively.

Questions

1 What is the diagnosis?
2 Give three useful investigations.
3 What is the treatment; how is this assessed?

Answer to case twenty-five

All these features are within the normal range. Children who 'bottom shuffle' often do not walk until relatively late, i.e. approximately 18 months.

A 3.1 kg baby of 30 hours of age is admitted to the special care baby unit having been noted to be breathless and reluctant to feed. The child is the third in the family. The two siblings are well and both parents are healthy, although a cousin of this child has phenylketonuria. Pregnancy and labour were normal and the Apgar score at 1 minute was 9. The baby was put to the breast in the labour room.

On examination, the child has mild central cyanosis and is breathless with a respiratory rate of 80 breaths/min. Femoral pulses are difficult to feel but present. Pulse rate is 200 beats/min. The liver edge is hard, palpable 4 cm below the costal margin. There is pitting oedema of the feet. There is a 3/6 systolic murmur in the pulmonary area.

The ECG shows sinus tachycardia and +90° axis and pulmonary venous congestion is noted on a chest x-ray.

Question

Give two likely diagnoses.

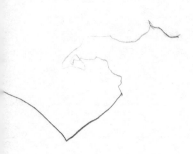

Answers to case twenty-six

1 At 7 minutes of age, the following should have been considered:

a blocked endotracheal tube.
b displaced endotracheal tube.
c presence of hypoglycaemia.
d blood gas analysis and possible bicarbonate infusion.
e repeat chest x-ray.
f transillumination of chest.

2 The child had Potter's syndrome. Points suggesting this are:

a failure to respond to the routine resuscitation because of hypoplastic lungs.
b low set ears.
c 'excessive skin'.

A 5-month-old male is admitted via casualty where he presented having had a fit. The parents state that he had not shown any change in his behaviour pattern that day.

The third of three children, he had had a normal delivery at term with good Apgar scores and was breast fed satisfactorily. He had smiled at 7 weeks and the parents were not concerned about the child's behaviour. The first child died aged 8 months at another hospital of an ill defined protracted illness. The second child is 7 years old and well. Father is a 34-year-old Irish diplomat and mother a 29-year-old Pakistani secretary. Both are healthy.

On examination, the child is on the 10th centile for length and weight and the 25th centile for head circumference. His skin looks very white and although his generalized fit has now terminated he is still having occasional repetitive twitching of both hands and the right eye. His head is almost bald, having just a little hair which is rather soft and springy. The temperature is 35.2°C. The rest of the examination adds little information. The child seems rather limp and unresponsive but he is post-ictal. However, 48 hours later there is little change and the nurses state that he is a poor feeder.

Neurological examination at this stage show him to be hypotonic with definite developmental delay and he does not smile.

Investigations

Haemoglobin	9.4 g/dl	LP	1 WBC, 1 RBC mm³,
White blood count	$8.1 \times 10^9/l$		no organisms are seen.
Normal differential			Glucose 3.1 mmol/l
Sodium	141 mmol/l		Protein 0.2 g/l
Potassium	4.3 mmol/l	Serum amino acids	Normal
Urea	3.0 mmol/l	Urine amino acids	Normal
HCO_3^-	28 mmol/l	Ammonia	25 μmol/l (21–47 μmol/l)
		Lactate	1 mmol/l (1.0–1.8)

Questions

1 Give the most likely diagnosis.
2 Give three useful investigations.
3 What is the prognosis?

Answers to case twenty-seven

1 *The girl has a dyshormonogenetic goitre. Points suggesting this are:*

a *signs of myxoedema.*
b *neck swelling increasing with age.*
c *sister similarly affected.*

Also consider juvenile hypothyroidism due to autoimmune thyroiditis. There is an increased familial incidence and would explain the family history.

2 *Useful investigations include:*

a *serum T_4.*
b *serum TSH.*
c *thyroid scan and perchlorate discharge.*
d *x-ray thoracic inlet.*
e *specific investigation for dyshormonogenetic enzyme defects.*

3 *Treat with thyroxine. Adequacy of treatment is assessed by suppressing TSH level to normal values.*

An 8-year-old boy is sent into hospital by his GP with a story that 1 month earlier he had seen the boy with fever and abdominal pain. The GP had diagnosed a urinary infection, confirmed by urine culture and had treated the boy with co-trimoxazole. Subsequently, the boy had improved with loss of pain and fever, but generally seemed rather depressed and, at the end of 2 weeks, the parents once more sought the GP's help because of his increasing depression. The GP reassured the parents that this was just a reaction to the febrile illness. Two weeks later the boy's mood has worsened. Previously, a very bright happy child doing well at school and a member of two football teams, he now merely sits and mopes.

On examination, he looks rather wasted and mother confirms he has lost 3 kg. His liver is palpable 2 cm below the costal margin. There are no other positive findings.

Investigations

Haemoglobin	12.3 g/dl
White blood count	$8.4 \times 10^9/l$
Electrolytes and creatinine	Normal
Liver function tests	Normal
Brucella titres	
Widal	
Paul-Bunnell	All negative
Viral titres	
Bone marrow	Normal
Urine culture	Normal
IVP	Normal
Skull x-ray	Normal
CAT scan (head)	Normal

Questions

1 What is the likely diagnosis?
2 What is the most important decision in management?

Answer to case twenty-eight

This child has the hypoplastic left heart syndrome. Points suggesting this are:
 a cyanosis.
 b early onset of heart failure.
 c compatible with other information given, e.g. pulmonary congestion.

Of course, the whole range of cyanotic congenital heart disease must be considered but transposition of the great arteries and infradiaphragmatic total anomalous pulmonary venous drainage would be reasonable alternatives.

A 7-month-old female infant is brought to outpatients by both parents. She is their first child. Father is 36 and a branch manager of a building society and mother a 28-year-old housewife. Both parents are very well and father knows of no family illness on his side but mother is an adopted child and unaware of her family background. The child had a forceps delivery at term for delay in the second stage of labour, but there were no other problems during pregnancy and delivery.

The parents complain that for the past 3–4 weeks the child had started screaming at tea times. On most evenings during that period she had seemed to become very agitated and while sitting in her high chair would throw herself forward towards the tray of her high chair and bang her head. When restrained she simply became more agitated.

On examination, the child is well grown and rather obese with dry eczematous patches on her back. She shows evidence of dermatographia and in this same area one or two rather pale patches of skin. Otherwise her appearance is quite normal. The respiratory and cardiovascular systems appear normal, but examination of the abdomen shows evidence of constipation. Her development is probably appropriate for a 7-month child.

Questions

1 Give the likely diagnosis.
2 Give two appropriate investigations.

Answers to case twenty-nine

1 The diagnosis here is Menkes' syndrome. Points suggesting this are:

a previous history of another child dying of an ill defined illness (in fact before Menkes' syndrome was first described).
b abnormal neurological state.
c anaemia/pale colour.

2 Useful investigations are:

a serum copper.
b serum caeruloplasmin.
c EEG.
d CAT scan.

3 Prognosis is poor, most dying in early infancy.

A 7-year-old boy is sent into hospital with a 2-week history of neurological deterioration. Symptoms began on Christmas Eve with a cough and a tendency to drop things. Over the Christmas period he had episodes of stumbling and soon afterwards there was a definite weakness of the legs and an inability to walk unaided. About 4 days prior to admission he had also developed rather bizarre, generalized twitching, randomly affecting his limbs, trunk and head. Both parents felt that the boy had had a very poor memory during this time and that his speech had become progressively slurred.

He is the third of five children, but all the siblings are well, as is his father. His mother, however, is a diabetic. The pregnancy and birth of this child were without incident and apart from all the usual childhood illnesses there had been no problems.

NOT Tub sclerosis

On examination, he is continually twitching and at times apparently writhing. He obeys some commands but his ability to speak or carry out a command is very limited. It is impossible to assess tone and power adequately, or the tendon reflexes, but the plantar responses are both flexor. The fundi are normal. Apart from a short systolic murmur all other systems appear normal.

Questions

1 What is the diagnosis?
2 Give three important investigations.

Answers to case thirty

1 This boy has a depressive psychosis. Points suggesting this are:

a the boy's general demeanour.
b lack of evidence for organic disease.

2 The important decision in management is to exclude all reasonable organic causes (e.g. myxoedema, Addison's disease, some degenerative disorders, drug ingestion and solvent abuse) and gain psychiatric help having made the positive step of informing parents and child of the lack of evidence for an organic basis to his illness.

An 8-month-old female infant is admitted with a history of malaise for at least 1 month. During that time the child has had episodes of fever and rashes. Intermittently there had been periods when the little girl had become miserable with swelling of the joints of her hands and feet.

Past medical history reveals that the child had been admitted at 4 months of age with diarrhoea and vomiting but also the mother felt that the child has had recurrent swelling of the joints of the hands and feet for some time. There is no relevant family history.

On examination, the child is pyrexial with swollen joints of both hands and feet. The child also appears unwilling to move her right hip. The child is generally miserable but there are no other abnormal findings.

Questions

1 Give the most likely diagnosis.
2 Give three useful investigations.

Answers to case thirty-one

1 This child is having salaam attacks caused by tuberose sclerosis. Points suggesting this are:

a description of attacks.
b presence of depigmented skin patches.

2 Useful investigations would be:

a EEG.
b skull x-ray.
c fundoscopy with mydriasis looking for phakomata.
d cerebral CAT scan.
e skin examination under Wood's light.

A 14-year-old girl is brought to hospital accompanied by the nurse of the public school which she attends. Until 3 weeks previously she had been perfectly well but had developed chicken pox which had run a mild course although she was kept isolated for 2 weeks. She remained well for 5 days but during the 48 hours prior to admission she had become increasingly delirious.

On examination, she is in grade II coma (Lovejoy scale), hyperventilating, with evidence of hypertonia and opisthotonos. Her pupils are widely dilated and the liver is palpable 2 cm below the costal margin.

Questions

1 What is the most likely diagnosis?
2 Give two important investigations.

Answers to case thirty-two

1 This child has subacute sclerosing panencephalitis (SSPE). Points suggesting this are:

a progressive neurological deterioration.
b presence of myoclonus.
c presence of choreoathetosis.
d past history of measles (i.e. one of the usual childhood illnesses).

Differential diagnoses include other gross degenerative disorders, an acute encephalitis, poisoning or a rapidly growing tumour.

2 Useful investigations to support the diagnosis of SSPE include:

a EEG.
b lumbar puncture.
c serum and CSF measles antibody titre.
d cerebral CAT scan.

A male infant, now 4 weeks of age, has developed an increased requirement for oxygen over the past 24 hours according to the transcutaneous oxygen electrode which is being used to monitor his progress. This has been confirmed by arterial blood gases.

He had been born at 30 weeks' gestation, the second of twins, weighing 1.2 kg. He had developed idiopathic respiratory distress syndrome (IRDS) by 30 minutes of age and at 12 hours of age required ventilation which had been maintained for $2\frac{1}{2}$ weeks. Subsequently he had been weaned down to 25% O_2 but during the last 24 hours this had needed to be increased to 30–35% O_2 and now he has had a brief apnoeic episode.

Both parents are young and well and this was the mother's first pregnancy. All had gone well until the spontaneous onset of labour at 30 weeks which had proceeded despite attempts to stop it. The first baby, a female weighing 1.1 kg had initially done well but had developed a spontaneous perforation of the ileum at 30 hours and had died during an operation to repair the defect.

A full examination of the baby reveals nothing new except for a mild increase in respiratory rate. At the onset of these problems, the previous day, a full septic screen had been performed and penicillin, gentamicin and aminophylline were given. Preliminary results of cultures are now available and all are negative.

Investigations

Haemoglobin	11.3 g/dl	HCO_3^-	19 mmol/l
White blood count	11.4×10^9/l	Urea	4.4 mmol/l
Neutrophils	50%	Bilirubin	Less than 20 μmol/l
Lymphocytes	45%	AST	4 U/l
Sodium	130 mmol/l	ALT	11 U/l
Potassium	4.1 mmol/l		

The chest x-ray shows some streaky shadowing in both lung fields but not consistent with pulmonary oedema. Several small cysts are present.

Questions

1 Give two most likely diagnoses.
2 Give three important steps in management.

Answers to case thirty-three

1 *This little girl has chronic juvenile polyarthritis. Points suggesting this are:*

a long-standing arthritis. b fever. c rash. d general misery.

Also to be considered are the various infective and post-infective causes of arthritis and arthralgia. Other autoimmune disorders such as systemic lupus erythematosus also enter the differential diagnosis.

2 *Useful investigations to clarify the diagnosis include:*

a ESR. b serum autoantibodies. c rheumatoid factor (IgM and IgG). d viral titres. e Widal and Brucella titres. f serum complement. g anticomplement activity. h C_3 degradation products.

which ones?

An 8-year-old boy is referred to outpatients with a 6-month history of frequent loose motions, approximately six times a day. There had been no associated blood but some mucus with the motions. During this period there has also been a tendency to soil. Bran added to the diet, suggested by the GP, had resulted in an initial improvement but after a few weeks there had been a relapse. The child's general health has otherwise been good, although an abscess, adjacent to his anus, had developed after he had been kicked on the bottom during a fight at school 8 months previously.

An only child, he was adopted by two young teachers, both well. He knows nothing of his real parents. He is an anxious child who is not getting on well at school and dislikes his teacher.

On examination, he is found to be thin but adequately grown, with stained teeth. There are no other abnormal findings on examination which included a rectal examination.

Investigations

Haemoglobin	7.6 g/dl	Potassium	3.8 mmol/l
White blood count	12.1 × 10⁹/l	HCO_3^-	29 mmol/l
Neutrophils	77%	Urea	2.5 mmol/l
Lymphocytes	10%	Protein	59 g/l
Eosinophils	8%	Iron	4.7 μmol/l (10.7–31.3 μmol/l)
Monocytes	5%	TIBC	43 μmol/l (26.3–83.8 μmol/l)
Stool culture and microscopy was negative.		B12	1000 pg/ml
		Folic acid	3.0 ng/ml
Sodium	134 mmol/l		

Questions

1 Give the likely diagnosis.
2 How would you confirm the diagnosis? Give two tests.

Answers to case thirty-four

1 *This girl has Reye's syndrome. Points suggesting this diagnosis are:*

a *onset following chicken pox.*
b *rapidly progressive encephalopathy.*
c *hepatomegaly.*

Other diagnoses to be considered are other causes of encephalopathy, viral meningo-encephalitis, a space occupying lesion and poisoning.

2 *Investigations useful in supporting the diagnosis of Reye's syndrome are:*

a *serum ammonia.*
b *blood sugar.*
c *liver enzymes.*
d *clotting studies.*
e *salicylate level.*

Also to be considered are lumbar puncture, viral titres, blood cultures and an EEG.

An 8-year-old boy is referred to hospital with a 3-month history of recurrent headache and vomiting. Prior to that time he had been very well. The attacks have no apparent precipitating or relieving factors and have occurred at various intervals. On occasion they have awakened the child from sleep. Between attacks he has been well and he has no other associated symptoms. There has been no abdominal pain.

He is the younger of the two children, having a sister aged 11 years. All members of the family are well. However, the parents have split up and father now lives two streets away with another woman.

On full examination of all systems, some blurring of the nasal optic disc margins is noted, with minimal clumsiness of the right hand.

Questions

1 What are the two most likely mechanisms to account for the problem?
2 What is the correct course of action?

Answers to case thirty-five

1 This baby has bronchopulmonary dysplasia. Points suggesting this are:

a birth weight 1.2 kg.
b increasing respiratory problems at 4 weeks.
c chest x-ray changes.
d previous artificial ventilation.

The Wilson–Mikity syndrome is a term usually reserved for persistent pulmonary dysfunction in infants who have breathed spontaneously. Septicaemia has obviously also been considered. A persistent ductus arteriosus and recurrent aspiration should be excluded.

2 The steps in management are:

a adequate respiratory support.
b adequate nutritional support is essential as satisfactory weight gain is critical for recovery.
c good general care, e.g. temperature control, to allow spontaneous resolution.
d parental support.

An 11-week-old female infant is admitted with her third attack of wheezing. She has had two previous admissions for similar episodes. The child had been quite well until 12 hours prior to admission when fairly abruptly she had developed persistent wheeze and cough during the night. She had been sent in by her GP when seen the next morning. Otherwise the child had no other symptoms. Mother had commented that even when well the child tended to have a rather rattly chest.

Pregnancy and labour had been normal but the child was small for dates and was a rather difficult feeder, tending to thrust her tongue and splutter on her feeds. However, her weight was now on the 10th centile. Both parents are in their early twenties. Father suffers from dermatitis herpetiformis and mother from asthma.

On examination, the child does not appear very ill but has mildly wheezy respiration. The respiratory rate is 45 breaths/min and there is minimal recession. Auscultation reveals widespread rhonchi of low pitch and a few crepitations at the right base.

Questions

1 Give three possible diagnoses.
2 Give six useful investigations.

Answers to case thirty-six

1 This boy is suffering from Crohn's disease. Points suggesting this are:

 a diarrhoea with relapsing course.
 b perianal abscess.
 c chronic anaemia.
 d low serum folate.

2 Investigations could include:

 a sigmoidoscopy and biopsy.
 b barium enema.
 c barium meal and follow-through.
 d ESR.

CASE THIRTY-NINE

A male infant, aged 3 weeks, is admitted with a history of poor feeding since birth. This had become much worse in the week prior to admission. His mother commented that he seemed unwilling to take milk, and for the last 48 hours had vomited all of his feeds. There had been some mild diarrhoea. He was a full term normal delivery, birth weight 3.4 kg and had transient tachypnoea for 12 hours after delivery. There is no relevant family history.

On examination, the child looks very ill, grossly malnourished and lethargic. His skin is mottled and he is still vomiting. There is impetigo on the tip of his nose and two of his toes. The liver is enlarged to 4 cm below the right costal margin. The scrotum and penis appear a little pigmented. (↑ ACTH)

dehydrated

Investigations

Sodium	106 mmol/l
Potassium	5.7 mmol/l
Urea	14.2 mmol/l
Creatinine	11.0 μmol/l
Glucose	3.4 mmol/l
Haemoglobin	16.4 g/dl
White blood count	12.9 $\times$ 10^9/l

An erect abdominal x-ray shows some bowel distension and fluid levels.

Questions

1 What is the diagnosis?
2 Give two important investigations.
3 Give three steps in treatment.

Answers to case thirty-seven

1 This boy had a posterior fossa tumour. Points suggesting this are:

a presence of headache and vomiting occurring during the day and waking him from sleep.
b presence of neurological signs.

Differential diagnosis includes other causes of raised intracranial pressure and possibly a psychological basis for his symptoms, although the latter is unlikely in view of the nocturnal headaches.

2 Investigations:

a skull x-ray.
b cerebral CAT scan.
c perhaps further fundoscopy using fluorescence to help evaluate the disc signs.
d CSF examination (may require craniotomy) including cytospin and identification of malignant cells.

An 8-month-old male infant is admitted with a 2-week history of vomiting. The vomiting has varied in severity during that time but each vomit has been large. On some days there have been six vomits, on others, just one. There is no relationship to feeds. He was seen by the GP at the beginning of the illness and promethazine was prescribed. On the day of admission there had been two vomits but the child now looked so pale and ill that the mother sought further help.

Birth history had been quite normal; mother is a 45-year-old housewife, father a 42-year-old coal miner. There is no relevant family illness.

On examination, he looks pale and ill, and about 10% dehydrated. The child is apyrexial and the only positive finding is a mass in the left loin.

Investigations

Haemoglobin	15.1 g/dl
White blood count	9.0×10^9/l
HCO_3^-	7.7 mmol/l
Potassium	5.3 mmol/l
Urea	21.0 mmol/l
Sodium	115 mmol/l
17-alpha-hydroxyprogesterone	1.4 mmol/l (normal)

Questions

1 What treatment is required now?
2 What is the diagnosis?
3 What is the most useful investigation?

Answers to case thirty-eight

1 This child suffered from a recurrent aspiration syndrome (gastro-oesophageal reflux). Other diagnoses considered were asthma, cystic fibrosis, tracheo-oesophageal fistula or other laryngo-tracheal anomaly and post-bronchiolitis syndrome. Points suggesting the true diagnosis are:

a recurrent attacks.
b feeding problems.
c chest signs.

2 Investigations which would help in the differential diagnoses include:

a chest x-ray.
b lateral x-ray of head and neck.
c barium swallow.
d sweat test.
e bronchoscopy.
f full blood count (looking for eosinophils).
g laryngoscopy.
h serum IgE.
i lung ventilation/perfusion scan.
j milk scan.

A 3-year-old girl presents to the outpatients department with a history of abdominal pain and vomiting recurring over the past 5 months. The symptoms have varied in frequency and duration and she has been constipated although her stools have been otherwise normal. For the past week she has been lethargic with a poor appetite. She has not been taking medication.

Her past medical history and family history are unremarkable.

On examination she is well grown. Her abdomen is slightly distended and a firm, non-tender liver is palpable 8 cm below the costal margin in the midclavicular line. There are no stigmata of chronic liver disease and no other masses are palpable.

The remainder of the physical examination is normal.

Investigations

Haemoglobin	9.7 g/dl
White cell count	7.4×10^9/l
Serum alphafetoprotein	90 000 μg/l (normal range less than 25 μg/l)

The following investigations were normal:
  a plasma electrolytes and urea.
  b plasma glucose, lactate, pyruvate, bicarbonate and uric acid after overnight fast.
  c red cell glycogen.
  d leucocyte 'glycogen pathway' enzymes.
  e fasting lipid profile.

Lymphocyte inclusions were not detected.

Questions

1 Give the likely diagnosis.
2 Give two further useful investigations.

Answers to case thirty-nine

1 This child was suffering from congenital adrenal hyperplasia. Points suggesting this diagnosis are:

a general condition.
b timing of onset.
c male phenotype.
d pigmented genitalia.
e electrolyte values.

2 Serum 17-alpha-hydroxyprogesterone measurement is the most important investigation in this situation but urinary steroid excretion and urinary electrolytes are also valuable.

3 The treatment required is intravenous administration of saline and dextrose, and the use of a glucocorticoid and a mineralocorticoid.
The differential diagnosis at the time of presentation included severe gastroenteritis, septicaemia and an obstructed urinary tract.

A male infant now 3 weeks old, weighs 1.6 kg. He had been born prematurely at 32 weeks' gestation weighing 1.5 kg. Delivery had been normal. After some initial weight loss he had regained his birth weight on day 10, but the subsequent gain had not been satisfactory.

The child's parents are deaf, having met at a school for the deaf. This is their first child and all had gone well until the sudden onset of labour at 32 weeks. He has required nasogastric tube feeding from the outset which has been well tolerated (200 ml/kg per day), although there has been some vomiting in the last 3 days.

On examination, there are no abnormal findings.

Questions

1 Give two possible diagnoses.
2 Give four helpful investigations.

Answers to case forty

1 The child needs immediate circulatory support. This was initially provided by an intravenous infusion of plasma, 20 ml/kg. Other measures to improve circulation and state of hydration would also have been useful.

2 He was suffering from bilateral pelviureteric junction obstruction. Points suggesting this are:

a general physical state with dehydration.
b loin mass (only unilateral on clinical examination).
c biochemical evidence of renal failure.

It is important to exclude urethral valves or an infected urinary tract.

3 Diagnosis was made with abdominal utrasound scan.

An 8-year-old boy is referred to hospital because he has recently developed a second facial palsy within 9 months. The initial episode had just resolved when the palsy on the other side occurred. With the second palsy there seemed to be more associated puffiness of the face. However, on the first occasion there were no other features. Mother reported that the boy's school were not pleased with his progress and that recently he had seemed very tired.

He had previously been entirely well, his only prior contact with hospital having been for a circumcision as an infant.

His parents are both 34 years old and well. There is one sibling aged 7 years who is well. There is no relevant familial illness.

On examination, he seems very nervous with a mild left facial palsy. The blood pressure is 150/110 mmHg but there are no other abnormal findings.

Questions

1 What is the most likely cause of the facial palsy?
2 Give three important investigations.

Answers to case forty-one

1 *This girl has a hepatoblastoma, although differentiation from hepatocellular carcinoma is not possible from the information given. Points suggesting the diagnosis are:*

  a abdominal distension.
  b malaise.
  c abdominal pain (unusual).
  d greatly raised alphafetoprotein.
  e normal results of investigations of storage disorders.

2 *A liver scan may be useful in defining the presence of a tumour as a filling defect. Hepatoarteriography may show displacement of normal vasculature and an abnormal tumour circulation. A percutaneous liver biopsy is not justified in view of the raised serum alphafetoprotein.*

CASE FORTY-FOUR

A 13-year-old boy, who is a known asthmatic, is admitted with an acute attack. He is seen by the doctor on duty who decides that the boy has mild symptoms and prescribes salbutamol inhalations to which the boy responds. Twelve hours later he has a recurrence of chest pain which he has had intermittently over the past 6 months.

At 6 years of age he had an operation for relief of a subvalvular aortic stenosis. Since that time he had generally been well, although his murmur persisted. During the 6 months prior to this admission he had complained intermittently of pains in his chest but this did not occur in relation to any particular event or activity.

On examination, his pulse is 90 beats/min, blood pressure 80/60 mmHg. The apex beat is thrusting and displaced to the 7th intercostal space in the anterior axillary line. There is a grade 5/6 ejection systolic murmur in the aortic area, radiating to the neck.

Questions

1 What is the likely significance of the chest pain?
2 Give three investigations required.

Answers to case forty-two

1 This boy was discovered to have a urinary tract infection. Other diagnoses considered in view of the lack of clinical signs were malabsorption, infection at another site or a possible metabolic disorder.

2 Investigations which may be useful in making the diagnosis include:

a urine culture (preferably obtained by suprapubic aspiration or clean catch).
b infection screen.
c full blood count.
d sweat test.
e stool for reducing substances.
f urine for reducing substances.
g capillary pH.
h serum and urine amino acids.
i serum lactate/pyruvate.
j serum ammonia.

Points in the history which suggest this diagnosis are:

a arrested weight gain.
b failure to tolerate feeds.
c lack of physical signs.

44 *Case Studies in Paediatrics*

A 12-year-old boy is sent into hospital following a consultant domiciliary visit, with a 4-week history of intermittent episodes of severe abdominal pain and weight loss. Appetite had been depressed during this time and nausea had accompanied the pain. He had bouts of mucousy diarrhoea but there had been no obvious blood present. There were no symptoms referable to any other system.

On examination, he looks ill and has obviously lost weight. His temperature is 37.5 °C. There is diffuse abdominal tenderness and rectal examination reveals loose mucousy stool which is positive for blood on testing. There are no other abnormal findings.

Investigations

Haemoglobin	8.7 g/dl
White blood count	12.1 × 10⁹/l
ESR	78 mm/h

Questions

1 What are the two most likely diagnoses?
2 Give the three most important investigations.
3 Give three steps in treatment.

Answers to case forty-three

1 The facial palsies were caused by this boy's hypertension. Points in the history which suggest this diagnosis are:

a two episodes of facial palsy separated in time.
b deterioration in general health.
c level of hypertension.

This is a recognized, though rare, cause of facial palsy. While in the ward it was recorded at a maximum of 200/140. Other possible diagnoses are Bell's palsy, polyradiculopathy (Guillain–Barré) and cerebral tumour (especially pontine). The time course made the latter unlikely.

2 Investigations of the hypertension include plasma urea, electrolytes and creatinine, abdominal x-ray, IVP, abdominal ultrasound scan, renal isotope scan and measurement of the glomerular filtration rate.

A boy aged 2 years 9 months is referred to hospital because of a series of upper respiratory tract infections. Various medications have been tried in the past, mainly antibiotics which were only of limited benefit. Salbutamol has been tried without help. There is no other symptomatology and pregnancy, birth and perinatal history were all unremarkable.

On examination, there are no abnormal findings. However, a poor view of the ears is obtained because of wax. The child's speech is limited and difficult to understand, and clinically the child's hearing appears impaired.

An audiogram shows the child to have a threshold for sound at 30 db.

Question

What is the most likely diagnosis for the speech defect and what initial therapy is required?

Answers to case forty-four

1 This boy had restenosed his aortic outflow tract and was suffering from angina. Points suggesting this diagnosis are:

a the history of the left ventricular outflow tract disease.
b history of recurrent pain.
c low systolic blood pressure for a boy of this age.

It is, of course, necessary to consider other causes of chest pain and in view of the asthmatic attack, pneumothorax must be excluded. Infection such as pneumonia or pericarditis need to be considered.

2 The ECG was useful, since it revealed ischaemic changes not previously present, as well as the signs of left ventricular hypertrophy. Chest x-ray and creatine phosphokinase were also useful. He subsequently underwent catheterization and aortic valve replacement.

Lisa, a 6-year-old girl, is referred by her school doctor because of increasing lethargy. She attends a school for the physically handicapped.

She has had other hospital attendances, originally presenting about 3 years previously with a history of clumsiness and was noted on examination to have signs compatible with a cerebellar disorder. Prominent blood vessels over her conjunctivae were also noted. A diagnosis was made and on the whole she had remained well until the 3 months prior to this admission. During this time she has become progressively more pale and tired, now tending to fall asleep in class.

On examination, she is pale but quite alert, orientated and able to answer questions freely. There is no fever. A smooth, firm mass extends from within the confines of the left costal margin to below the umbilicus and into the loin. The signs of her other disease process remain unchanged and there are no additional findings.

Investigations

Haemoglobin	7.5 g/dl
White blood count	7.3×10^9/l
Normal differential	

Questions

1 What was the original diagnosis?
2 What is the underlying process predisposing to the formation of the mass?
3 Give four investigations.

Answers to case forty-five

1 This boy was in fact eventually diagnosed as having ulcerative colitis although clinically a diagnosis of Crohn's disease was felt to be more likely. Points suggesting the diagnosis are:

a fever.
b general malaise, weight loss and abdominal pain.
c diarrhoea with mucus and blood.
d anaemia.
e raised ESR.

2 Diagnosis was actually made by sigmoidoscopy and biopsy, with further information obtained from a barium enema. Barium meal and follow-through would have been useful if the previous investigations had been negative. Microscopy and culture of the stools were negative, excluding an infective cause.

3 This boy was transfused, given a low residue diet and treated with a combination of salazopyrine and steroids. In fact he failed to make any satisfactory long term response and came to surgery some months later.

An 18-month-old boy is referred because of persistent drowsiness. On close questioning it appears that for the past few weeks he has tended to drift off into a deep sleep during the day even while occupied in some activity. The passage from waking to sleeping is fairly quick and once asleep he can be roused but with some difficulty. His parents feel at times during an attack he has looked a little blue. Otherwise he has been well apart from upper respiratory tract infections and a tendency to snore at night.

His parents are both in their early thirties and are well, although father had suffered from severe asthma as a child. There are two other siblings, both older, who are well.

Pregnancy, birth and perinatal history are all normal.

On examination, he seems well with normal development and growth. His chest appears a little asymmetrical with a slight prominence of the right sternal edge. Examination of the cardiovascular system reveals a prominent second heart sound. Examination of the respiratory system appears normal except for very large tonsils. There are no other abnormal findings.

Investigations

Haemoglobin	14.1 g/dl
White blood count	6.4×10^9/l
Sodium	132 mmol/l
Potassium	4.1 mmol/l
Urea	4.6 mmol/l
HCO_3^-	27 mmol/l

Po_2 7.9 kPa, HCO_3^- 27 mmol/l, pH 7.33 – at rest
Po_2 7.3 kPa, HCO_3^- 28 mmol/l, pH 7.31 – during an attack

Questions

1 What is the mechanism for the drowsiness?
2 What is the treatment?

Answers to case forty-six

Once the wax was removed it became clear that this boy's problem was chronic serous otitis media or glue ear. Points suggesting this diagnosis are:

    a chronic upper respiratory tract infections.
    b poor speech.
    c impaired hearing.

This had almost certainly been present for a considerable length of time and as a result had impaired his language development. He was treated with nasal decongestants for a short period before having grommets inserted.

48 Case Studies in Paediatrics

A 36-hour-old male infant is transferred to the special care baby unit because of failure to pass meconium and abdominal distension. The infant has also started to vomit after his last two feeds. These vomits were bile stained.

There had been a normal pregnancy and delivery but the child had been in poor condition at birth with an Apgar score of 4 at 1 minute. He responded to facial oxygen and had an Apgar score of 9 at 5 minutes. Urine was passed normally and initially he had fed well but subsequently had become rather reluctant.

On examination now, he is apyrexial but appears floppy with obvious distension of the abdomen. The anus is normal and the rectum is empty on digital examination. Following the latter procedure, the child passes some very thick meconium including a small plug. Twelve hours later the distension is less but has not resolved following passage of a little more meconium.

Investigations

Haemoglobin	12.3 g/dl
White blood count	6.3×10^9/l
Neutrophils	50%
Lymphocytes	50%

There is marked toxic granulation.

Sodium	129 mmol/l
Potassium	4.3 mmol/l
Urea	3.6 mmol/l
HCO_3^-	21 mmol/l

An abdominal x-ray shows generally distended bowel at least to the descending colon, and there are multiple fluid levels on the erect film. The abdominal x-ray taken after passage of meconium shows air to the rectum.

Question

Give the three most likely diagnoses and indicate an investigation to confirm each proposed diagnosis.

Answers to case forty-seven

1 This little girl has ataxia telangiectasia (Louis-Bar syndrome): an inherited cerebellar ataxia associated with telangiectasia of the whole bulbar conjunctivae and sometimes more extensive telangiectasis. Points suggesting this diagnosis are:

a cerebellar signs.
b conjunctival telangiectasia.
c anaemia (arisen secondary to the malignancy).

Other associated features are variable immune deficiencies and increased chromosomal breakage. The latter is responsible for an increased incidence of malignancy in this condition and here has produced a lymphoma. The mass was expected to be a spleen but in fact turned out to be a huge mass of lymph nodes. Numerous relevant investigations are possible and include:

a urea and electrolytes.
b creatinine clearance.
c urinary VMA.
d abdominal and chest x-rays.
e IVP.
f abdominal ultrasound scan.
g laparotomy.
h bone marrow.
i bone scan.

A 6-week-old male infant is admitted as a feeding problem. The history is non-specific although the child had invariably been a poor feeder during the first 6 weeks of his life. There were no other complaints.

The parents were both in their mid-thirties and had two other children, both girls, who were well. The pregnancy and birth history of this child were unremarkable.

On examination, the child is odd in appearance with a rather wizened face and many creases around the eyes. His hair is thin and sparse. Height and head circumference are on the 25th centile but weight is below the 3rd. There are no other specific findings. He is admitted for a few days to be investigated and it is noted that each evening his temperature rises and he seems agitated. During these times his skin is hot but he does not sweat.

On the fifth night his temperature reaches 40 °C and he has a generalized convulsion. Lumbar puncture is performed with normal findings.

Questions

1 What is the cause of the fit? Give two investigations which are immediately required.
2 What do you think is the most likely diagnosis?

Answers to case forty-eight

1 The problem here is alveolar hypoventilation secondary to severe upper airway obstruction by the tonsils and adenoids. Points suggesting this diagnosis are:

a episodes of drowsiness associated with cyanosis.
b presence of very large tonsils producing snoring at night.
c evidence of right ventricular hypertrophy and pulmonary hypertension.
d hypoxia with a compensated respiratory acidosis.

2 Tonsillectomy.

A female infant is born at term after a normal pregnancy and delivery, birth weight 3.4 kg. At birth an abnormal facies is noted consisting of a short philtrum and low-set ears. Other dysmorphic findings are a right talipes equinovarus and a single umbilical artery. Cyanotic episodes and jitteriness are noted at 3 days of age and at 8 days she has several brief focal fits, which are treated with anticonvulsants. A cardiac murmur is also noted at this time and cardiac catheterization is performed showing a patent ductus arteriosus. At 6 months of age, she is failing to thrive and over the next year has numerous admissions for respiratory infections and pneumonia.

Questions

1 What is the diagnosis to associate all these features?
2 What is the cause of the fits?
3 Is there an associated chromosomal abnormality? What is the inheritance?

**Answer to
case forty-nine**

This child was septicaemic, confirmed by blood culture. A paralytic ileus is not uncommon in neonates who are ill from any cause. Points suggesting this diagnosis are:

a bile-stained vomiting and failure to pass meconium.
b hypotonia.
c presence of toxic granulation.

Other possibilities are Hirschsprung's disease which would require biopsy for confirmation, and meconium ileus which would be confirmed (and possibly treated) by Gastrografin enema. Further confirmation of cystic fibrosis would of course require a subsequent sweat test.

A 3-year-old child is admitted to hospital with a 3-week history of increasing sleeplessness, irritability and episodes of hyperextension of her neck. Initially she was thought to have a behaviour problem and was given prochlorperazine by the GP. Following two doses of this, she was given 60 mg promethazine on 3 days in succession. Persistence of the symptoms led her parents to seek further advice.

On examination, she is found to be irritable with opisthotonus. Examination of her cranial nerves is normal and there is no papilloedema. Her reflexes are difficult to elicit, but she has increased tone in all four limbs. The spleen and liver are just palpable. She is treated with benzhexol with some initial apparent improvement. The following day she is still pyrexial, with a stiff neck and a positive Kernig's sign. A lumbar puncture is performed, which is a traumatic tap, and bloody CSF is obtained. A CAT scan is also performed which is normal. Following this, her status improves and she is discharged.

However, she is readmitted 3 days later unable to bear weight on her legs because of weakness. On examination, her legs are hypotonic, reflexes in the legs are absent and the plantar responses are flexor. Her arms are normal. A lumbar puncture is repeated, but no CSF is obtained. The bladder is found to be distended.

Questions

1 What is the differential diagnosis?
2 Name five investigations that would aid the diagnosis.
3 What is the significance of the drugs given?

Answers to case fifty

1 Fever is almost certainly the cause of the fit but it is important to look for other possibilities and serum calcium and glucose should be measured now although magnesium, ammonia, pyruvate and lactate are all relevant. Further cultures looking for infection are also justified.

2 The actual diagnosis here and the cause of the fever is ectodermal dysplasia, a sex-linked recessive disorder affecting ectodermal structures. There are no sweat glands, hair is sparse, skin is dry and, later, teeth are very malformed. Particular care is required at times of fever and during very hot weather. Points suggesting this diagnosis are:

a male infant.
b thin sparse hair.
c episodes of fever.
d lack of sweating.

A 4-year-old boy is seen because of delayed milestones. His birth and neonatal history were normal. However, he sat at 12 months, stood at 15 months and walked at 19 months. He used a few words with meaning at 12 months, was dry by day at 2 years and by night at 3 years.

Both parents are well and there is no family history of illness. There are two siblings, a boy of 6 years and a girl of 3 years, both well.

On examination, he has a waddling gait with lordosis. The deltoid and calf muscles appear hypertrophied. The tendon reflexes are slow, except for ankle jerks which are normal. The muscles are not tender.

Questions

1 What is the differential diagnosis?
2 What three investigations would you suggest?
3 Would the presence of myoglobinuria help with the diagnosis?

Answers to case fifty-one

1 DiGeorge syndrome (III and IV pharyngeal pouch syndrome). Important features are: abnormal facies, convulsions (hypocalcaemic), heart disease, and frequent infective episodes.

2 Hypocalcaemia.

3 Normal chromosomes. Sporadic occurrence, but twice as frequent in males than in females.

A 2-year-old boy was referred from the eye hospital, where he had been admitted for correction of strabismus. Preoperatively he was found to have a haemoglobin of 4.0 g/dl and he was ketotic. His mother was of low intelligence and had fed him only on milk since birth.

He was born at term after a normal pregnancy, birth weight 3.3 kg. There were no neonatal problems. He walked at 2 years, was not yet dry and had a few words only at the time of assessment. No other history was available from her.

On examination, he was very withdrawn and clinging. He was pale with a few bruises on the limbs. There was a soft systolic ejection murmur at the left sternal edge and the liver was just palpable below the right costal margin. There was a marked convergent squint, with a rapid pendular nystagmus and intermittent head jerking.

Investigations

Haemoglobin   4.5 g/dl
A hypochromic film was noted.
Serum iron   1.9 μmol/l
Bone age   1 year 10 months
There was a low serum alanine and high levels of branched chain amino acids.

Questions

1 What is his neurological condition?
2 What is the aetiology and prognosis?
3 What is the cause of the abnormal serum amino acids?

**Answers to
case fifty-two**

1 This child had a spinal (lumbar) astrocytoma. CSF was not obtained because of anatomical distortion by the tumour.
Other diagnoses to consider are:

a post-infectious polyneuritis.
b meningitis.
c poliomyelitis.
d cord compression (abscess, haematoma, leukaemic infiltrate).
e tuberculous meningitis.

2 Five investigations which would aid diagnosis are:

a cisternal puncture for CSF.
b spinal CAT scan.
c viral serology.
d urinary vanillylmandelic acid level (VMA).
e bone marrow aspiration.

3 A 'red herring' initially, but they probably aggravated her neurological status.

A 12-year-old boy was admitted following an episode of haematemesis associated with epigastric pain. He had come to the UK one month prior to this admission, from Turkey, where he had been seen at 6 years of age for jaundice and abdominal swelling. He had been treated with an unknown medication and the swelling had resolved. A further episode had occurred 3 months prior to this admission while in Munich.

Past medical history: normal pregnancy and delivery. No neonatal problems. No other serious illnesses.

Family history: both parents well, unrelated and now separated. A sibling had died in Turkey at 7 years of age of unknown cause.

On examination, he was afebrile, lethargic and pale. Pulse 90 beats/min, blood pressure 110/60 mmHg, with good peripheral perfusion. The chest was clear. The liver was just palpable and the spleen was enlarged 5 cm below the left costal margin. Examination of the cranial nerves was normal. There was some generalized hypertonicity particularly on the right but muscle power and reflexes were normal and the plantar responses were flexor. Fine hand control was normal. Urine testing showed mild glycosuria.

Questions

1 What is the immediate problem?
2 What is the underlying problem?
3 What investigations would confirm this?
4 What therapeutic procedures would you initiate and how would you monitor the success of these?

Answers to case fifty-three

1 He has classical Duchenne muscular dystrophy. His initial history is normal, with appropriate development. The gradual deterioration with abnormal gait, muscle hypertrophy and slowing of reflexes is typical.
Also consider:

a polymyositis (although the muscles are usually painful).
g glycogen storage disease (McArdle's), although rare at this age. ~~Type I (Pompe)~~
c Kugelberg–Welander (juvenile spinal muscular atrophy).
d myotonia congenita.

2 Serum creatine phosphokinase level; electromyography; muscle biopsy.

3 Myoglobinuria is present in Duchenne muscular dystrophy and McArdle's disease.

A 10-year-old Caucasian girl presents with a 4-day history of increasing cough, fever, malaise and pleuritic pain. On the day of admission she is also experiencing pain in her right elbow, which has become swollen and hot over the past 3 days. She has also had recurrent episodes of malaise and aphthous ulcers, usually once or twice per month. She has had one previous hospital admission for appendicitis.

Both parents are well. Her father is a sewage worker and her mother is a housewife. There are three older siblings, all well. Her father keeps pigeons and there are about 30 cages in the back garden.

The neonatal history is normal. There have been no episodes of wheeze or dyspnoea in the past.

On examination, she has coarse rhonchi in her right lower lobe and a hot, swollen tender elbow. There are herpetic spots on her upper lip.

Questions

1 What is her present illness?
2 What is the underlying illness?
3 What treatment would you suggest?

Answers to case fifty-four

1 Spasmus nutans.

2 It is found at this age secondary to social deprivation and perhaps secondary to insufficient exposure to light. It often resolves spontaneously, but the child may develop other long-term problems, both physical and psychological, as a result of this deprivation.

3 Starvation.

A 4-month-old boy is admitted for investigation of failure to thrive. His mother has recently noted periods of acute dyspnoea and a rapid heart beat, often in association with going 'off colour'. Her other child has Down's syndrome and he also has blue spells, but because the baby's episodes were much milder, she had not worried about them initially.

There were no perinatal problems and apart from the sibling, there was no abnormal family history.

On examination, you find minimal cyanosis, a slightly enlarged liver and on auscultation of the heart there is a triple rhythm, with a widely split second sound and a soft systolic ejection murmur at the left sternal edge.

Questions

1 What is the probable diagnosis?
2 What would the ECG look like?
3 What treatment would you suggest?

Answers to case fifty-five

1 Bleeding oesophageal varices.

2 Wilson's disease. Points suggesting this are:
  a evidence of portal hypertension.
  b family history.
  c neurological signs.
  d glycosuria.

  Hydatid disease should be considered.

3 Investigations:

  a gastroscopy and/or barium swallow.
  b serum caeruloplasmin.
  c 24-hour urinary copper.
  d liver scan and liver biopsy (for histology and liver copper assay)
  e liver function tests.
  f slit lamp examination of the eyes.
  g urinary amino acids.
  h clotting studies.

4 a Immediate treatment: blood transfusion, vitamin K, fresh frozen plasma, neomycin, lactulose, Sengstaken tube.
  b Long term treatment: penicillamine pyridoxine, 24-hour urinary copper, which should increase after appropriate therapy.

A 1-year-old Italian boy presents with a 2-day history of vomiting and diarrhoea. He is treated with clear oral fluids and normal feeds are reintroduced over 3 days. However, the diarrhoea returns with the reintroduction of solid food. He loses weight and remains rather irritable.

Past medical history: born at 42 weeks' gestation, birth weight 3.2 kg. He was breast fed for 9 weeks and then with 'humanized' cows' milk. Solids were introduced at 4 months and 'door step' cows' milk at 12 months. He was fully immunized.

On examination, his height is on the 75th centile but weight is on the 30th centile. His development is normal; however, he is generally rather wasted and there are several small areas of ecchymosis on his limbs and trunk.

Investigations

Haemoglobin	13.1 g/dl
PCV	0.4
MCV	76 fl
White cell count	16.6×10^9/l

Poikylocytosis and acanthocytes are noted on the film and there are 2% reticulocytes. There are low levels of IgG, IgM and serum folate.

Questions

1 What is the diagnosis? Give a differential diagnosis.
2 What three further investigations are necessary?
3 What is the correct treatment?
4 What other manifestations of this disease will appear later?

Answers to case fifty-six

1 Pneumonia and osteomyelitis or septic arthritis. Points suggesting these diagnoses:

a cough, fever.
b pleuritic pain.
c herpes labialis.
d signs in chest and elbow.

2 Cyclical neutropenia, immunodeficiency.
An underlying immunological defect is suggested by the recurrent episodes of aphthous ulceration.

3 Systemic antibiotics (including a penicillinase resistant penicillin e.g. flucloxacillin as Staphylococcus aureus *is the most common organism in all age groups). Also consider H. influenzae and S. pneumoniae.*
Treatment with androgens and long term antibiotics (e.g. co-trimoxazole) may help prevent recurrent infection.

A 15-month-old Caucasian girl presents with a 10-day history of puffy eyes and gradually increasing abdominal distension. She is brought to hospital because of sudden onset of fever. She has previously been well and had no neonatal problems. Both parents have hay fever and a sibling has asthma. She has recently had a measles inoculation with a febrile reaction, but had recovered.

On examination, she has slight facial oedema and a tender, distended abdomen. She is febrile, temperature 38.5 °C, and has poor peripheral perfusion. There are no rashes.

Questions

1 What is the likely diagnosis?
2 What five investigations would you suggest immediately?
3 What is the cause of the low serum sodium concentration in this condition?
4 What three therapeutic steps would you initiate?

**Answers to
case fifty-seven**

1 This boy has Ebstein's anomaly. This is suggested by:

  a tachycardic episodes (supraventicular tachycardia) in association with cyanosis.
  b enlarged liver.
  c abnormal heart sounds.

  An AV canal is less likely to cause tachypnoea and tachycardia at this age. Congenital tricuspid incompetence is possible but is rare. Endocardial fibroelastosis is unlikely to produce acute episodes of failure.

2 Tall P waves (P pulmonale); right bundle branch block; normal or prolonged P-R interval; Wolff–Parkinson–White syndrome present in 30%.

3 a Surgical: this is difficult with a high mortality:
    i palliative – a Glenn operation or a Blalock–Taussig shunt.
    ii prosthetic tricuspid valve.
  b Medical: treat the failure with diuretics (thiazide or frusemide) and digoxin. Treat the arrhythmia with prophylactic propranolol or acutely with verapamil, practolol, digoxin or DC shock.

An 18-month-old Bangladeshi girl is referred with a 3-month history of enlarging breasts. There has been no galactorrhoea and no menses.

The neonatal period was normal. She was bottle fed from birth and although solid foods were introduced at 2 months, she takes these very reluctantly and in small amounts. Her parents give a history of her having recurrent bouts of diarrhoea for the past year and there had been some slowing of her weight gain over the past 3 months.

Both parents are well. A sibling, a boy of 6 months, is also well.

Development: sat at 6 months, crawled at 8 months, walked at 15 months and now has several words.

On examination, the weight and height are on the 1st centile and there is definite breast tissue palpable bilaterally.

Questions

1 What three other physical signs would you look for?
2 What is the likely diagnosis?
3 Give a differential diagnosis.
4 What investigations are necessary to establish or exclude the diagnosis?
5 What is the likely outcome?

Answers to case fifty-eight

1 *He is suffering from abetalipoproteinaemia. Typical features are the acanthocytosis, ecchymoses and diarrhoea (from steatorrhoea).*
Other diagnoses to consider are:

 a *coeliac disease.*
 b *giardiasis.*
 c *cows' milk protein intolerance, secondary to gastroenteritis.*
 d *intestinal lymphangiectasia.*

2 *Lipid immunoelectrophoresis, small bowel biopsy, measure serum cholesterol, phospholipid and triglycerides.*

3 *There is no specific treatment but a low fat intake and supplements of medium chain triglycerides may help. Fat soluble vitamins are necessary.*

4 *Ataxia; retinitis pigmentosa.*

A 7-year-old Caucasian girl is referred with abdominal pain and pyrexia following an upper respiratory tract infection. She has had intermittent abdominal pain, particularly right sided, for the past year.

Past medical history: born at 32 weeks' gestation. She developed the respiratory distress syndrome requiring respiratory support for 1 week, and had phototherapy for jaundice. She was breast fed initially, but later was fed with 'humanized' milk after discharge at 5 weeks of age. There had been no other illnesses subsequently, apart from repeated nose bleeds.

Her father is well, although he had an abdominal operation at 10 years of age. Mother has cirrhosis. A sibling, a boy of 3 months, had died 2 years previously with pneumonia.

On examination, she is febrile, her chest is clear, her liver is just palpable and non-tender, and the spleen is palpable 2 cm below the left costal margin.

Investigations

Haemoglobin	9.1 g/dl
Reticulocyte count	6%
MCHC	41.0%
MCH	3.16 pg
MCV	90 fl
Urea	3.0 mmol/l
Sodium	145 mmol/l
Potassium	5.0 mmol/l
Glucose	5.1 mmol/l

Questions

1 What is the diagnosis?
2 What two investigations would confirm this?
3 What other investigation is required?

Answers to case fifty-nine

1 Nephrotic syndrome complicated by peritonitis.

2 a Haemoglobin, and packed cell volume.
b Electrolytes.
c Serum albumin.
d 24 hour urinary albumin.
e Peritoneal tap for microscopy and culture.

3 Dilutional hyponatraemia due to lipid phase displacement.

4 Plasma expansion with plasma or albumin; intravenous penicillin; prednisolone.

A 42-week gestation baby is born after a normal pregnancy and delivery. She is noted to be floppy at birth, does not cry and there is poor facial movement. Although remaining floppy, she feeds adequately and gains weight. Solids are introduced at 5 months. At 10 months of age she is able to close her mouth, support her head and pull to sitting. She can sit alone for several minutes and has one or two words. She is referred for correction of club feet.

Father is well but mother has episodes of tiredness and weakness. A sibling has Down's syndrome.

On examination, she has an expressionless face, a high arched palate and bilateral talipes equinovarus. There is a strabismus and a soft systolic ejection murmur at the left sternal edge.

Investigations

CPK 179 units/l; EMG shows patchy myopathy in the tibialis anterior. Mother's EMG also shows a marked myopathy.

Questions

1 What is the likely diagnosis?
2 What treatment would you suggest?
3 What is the prognosis?

Answers to case sixty

1 a Hair: pubic, axillary and generalized.
  b Abnormal genitalia.
  c Pigmented areas.

2 Premature thelarche.

3 a True isosexual precocious puberty due to autonomous gonadatrophin production. Idiopathic in 80% of females. Also consider hypothalamic disease or pituitary disease (craniopharyngioma, post-traumatic or infective hydrocephalus, tuberose sclerosis, McCune – Albright polyostotic fibrous dysplasia, hamartoma) or gonadotrophin-producing tumour.
  b Precocious pseudo-puberty due to autonomous secretion of sex hormones from adrenal or gonadal tumour, or congenital adrenal hyperplasia.
  c Ingestion of exogenous hormones, e.g. contraceptive pill.

4 Bone age. If this is normal there is no need to perform further investigations at this stage. Close follow-up is essential. If bone age advance is present or develops, the following investigations are indicated:

  a serum LH, FSH, prolactin levels, both resting and stimulated.
  b urinary oestriols.
  c serum 17-alpha-hydroxyprogesterone.
  d serum T_4 and TSH.
  e x-ray skull and long bones.

5 Isolated thelarche has a good prognosis.

A 9-year-old black girl first presents with a 3-day history of pyrexia, vomiting and jaundice. Infectious hepatitis is diagnosed.

Investigations at this time

Plasma bilirubin	40 μmol/l
ALT	80 U/l
AST	43 U/l
PTT	13 seconds

Hepatitis B antigen (Hb_s Ag) positive

She recovers from this episode and remains symptom free for a year. She is admitted again because of persistent hepatomegaly.

Investigations on this occasion

ALT	114 U/l
AST	48 U/l
Albumin	33 g/l
Globulin	64.5 g/l

Autoantibodies negative

Alpha-1 antitrypsin phenotype normal

A liver biopsy shows chronic inflammatory cell infiltrate in portal tracts, fibroblastic proliferation and distortion of hepatic lobular architecture.

Questions

1 What is the probable diagnosis?

She is treated with corticosteroids; however, she continues to have hepatomegaly with jaundice and her liver function tests deteriorate.

Questions

2 Why did corticosteroids not improve her condition?
3 What would you suggest treating her with now?

She is readmitted a year later with a haemoglobin of 6.5 g/dl, PCV 0.35 and MCH 29 pg.

Questions

4 What is the cause of these abnormal values?
5 What investigations would you suggest for the cause of these?

Answers to case sixty-one

1 Hereditary spherocytosis. This was inherited from her father as suggested by his splenectomy at 10 years of age. Elliptocystosis is also possible. She has had episodes of abnormal pain from her gall stones. Her low haemoglobin, raised reticulocyte count, and raised MCHC are typical of spherocytosis.

2 a Film for spherocytosis.
  b Red cell fragility.

3 Cholecystogram or abdominal ultrasound.

A 32-week gestation female infant is admitted to the special care baby unit following fetal distress and birth asphyxia. Although she breathes spontaneously after resuscitation, she develops recurrent generalized convulsions at 24 hours of age. A cerebral CAT scan shows opacification of the ventricles which is enhanced with contrast medium. Her fits are controlled with phenobarbitone, and her subsequent progress is uncomplicated.

She is discharged home at 8 weeks feeding well. Her development is normal until 6 months when she develops recurrent crying episodes followed by sudden bouts of flexion of the trunk and head, and extension of the arms. These occur five to six times per day. An EEG is performed, which shows irregular spike and wave forms occurring at 2 cycles/ec.

On examination, her head circumference is at the lower limit of normal. No other neurological abnormalities are noted.

Questions

1 What is the diagnosis?
2 What is the appropriate treatment?
3 Is there a connection with the birth history?

Answers to case sixty-two

1 Congenital dystrophia myotonica. Initial signs of the disease are variable and myotonia often tends to develop later. Expression in the neonatal period tends to reflect inheritance from the mother.

2 Treat talipes appropriately. The child may need special schooling for physical and mental handicap, family support and genetic counselling.

3 Often improves in childhood, but deterioration occurs in adulthood, with increasing debility and death from pneumonia or heart failure by the fifth or sixth decade.

A 4-year-old Caucasian boy presents with sudden onset of high fever and he then develops a diffuse erythematous rash over 24 hours. The conjunctivae are inflamed, the palms and soles become swollen and erythematous and he experiences mild, flitting joint pains.

On examination, in addition to the above signs, he has mouth ulcers and cervical lymphadenopathy.

He remains febrile for 2 weeks, but his illness resolves without any sequelae.

Investigations

Haemoglobin	10.8 g/dl
White cell count	14 × 10⁹/l
Neutrophils	40%
Lymphocytes	50%
ALT	60 U/l
AST	70 U/l

Bilirubin less than 17 μmol/l. There is moderate proteinuria.

Questions

1 What is the likely diagnosis?
2 What other investigation is important (may need to be repeated)?
3 What is the prognosis?
4 What is the correct treatment?

Answers to case sixty-three

1 Chronic active hepatitis.

2 Her chronic active hepatitis was due to HBₛAg positive hepatitis. Corticosteroids are less effective in this type of chronic active hepatitis, or may be required in a larger dose.

3 Azathioprine, in addition to corticosteroids.

4 Oesophageal varices. Consider also a Coombs' positive haemolytic anaemia.

5 Barium meal and/or oesophagoscopy; Coombs' test; measure serum haptoglobins.

An 8-year-old boy presents with wasting of the muscles of his legs and talipes. A left tibialis anterior tendon transplant had been performed but unfortunately 3 years post operatively he fell and fractured his right femur. His gait gradually became more abnormal and he was seen to drag his foot. Recently he developed recurrent episodes of cough at night and occasional dyspnoea, especially in association with exercise.

Past medical history: born at 38 weeks' gestation by elective Caesarean section for maternal diabetes. Birth weight 4.5 kg. He was polycythaemic at birth and required a plasma exchange transfusion. He was jittery for the first 48 hours, but no fits occurred. He fed well and no further problems developed.

Family history: father 32, a milkman, has hayfever. Mother, 30, is a diabetic and there are three siblings, triplets, by mother's previous marriage who are healthy.

On examination, he is a thin child with a hyperexpanded chest. There is distal wasting of the muscles of the hand and distal muscles of the legs, with decreased power. The tendon reflexes are absent and there is also mild patchy sensory loss with 'glove stocking' distribution noted in the legs. There is minimally decreased visual acuity.

Investigations

CSF – 2 lymphocytes/mm^3, protein 0.3 g/l, sugar 3.5 mmol/l.

Questions

1 What is the diagnosis?
2 What investigations would you perform?
3 What is the inheritance in this case?

Answers to case sixty-four

1 Intraventricular haemorrhage.

2 Infantile spasms. (A variant EEG may be obtained which is not classical hypsarrhythmia.) The clinical description of attacks is typical of this disorder.

3 ACTH, prednisolone or dexamethasone: nitrazepam.

4 Yes. Infantile spasms represent a non-specific reaction to a variety of insults including perinatal birth injury or asphyxia. Other causes include neontal meningitis, phenylketonuria, tuberose sclerosis, neurofibromatosis, central nervous system congenital malformations, congenital infection or intrauterine growth retardation.

A 5-year-old girl is admitted with a 2-month history of polyuria and nocturia, but not enuresis. She has polydipsia and mother has often found her drinking from the bathroom tap. She is not eating as well as usual and has in fact lost 2 kg in 2 months.

Past medical history: born at 36 weeks' gestation by Caesarean section for pre-eclampsia. Birth weight 2.1 kg. She had asymptomatic hypoglycaemia and was treated with an intravenous dextrose infusion for 48 hours. Subsequently she was breast fed and developed normally. Cows' milk was introduced at 2 months but solids were not introduced until 7 months. She had two admissions to hospital at 3 and 4 years of age for abdominal pain, although no cause was found.

Family history: mother 24, epileptic, treated with phenytoin; father, 26, a lorry driver. There is a 3-year-old brother who is well.

On examination, she is thin, but not ill. Blood pressure 100/60 mmHg. There are no murmurs and her chest is clear. Her liver is palpable 4 cm below the costal margin. There is a slight proptosis. However, the fundi are normal. There are no other neurological signs.

Questions

1 What is the cause of her presenting complaint?
2 What is the underlying problem?
3 What three investigations would you suggest to establish your diagnosis?

Answers to case sixty-five

1 Kawasaki's disease (acute febrile mucocutaneous lymph node syndrome). Features suggesting this diagnosis are:

a fever.
b conjunctivitis.
c mouth ulcers.
d inflammation of palms and soles.
e exanthema.
f cervical lymphadenopathy.
g arthralgia.

In fact, five of the above criteria are sufficient to make the diagnosis.
The differential diagnosis includes:

a Stevens–Johnson syndrome.
b viral illness.
c scarlet fever.
d Reiter's syndrome.

2 ECG. Coronary arteritis is present in 50% of cases. The coronary angiogram is abnormal in 30–60% of cases.

3 There is 2% mortality from a coronary aneurysm, cardiac failure or coronary thrombosis. Death usually occurs within 2 months of the onset of the illness.

4 There is no accepted treatment. Antibiotics have not been associated with clinical improvement and neither corticosteroids nor aspirin affect the duration of fever. Drugs that reduce platelet stickiness, e.g. aspirin may decrease the incidence of coronary thrombosis.

A 2-year-old West Indian boy is admitted with a 4-week history of cough, malaise, fever and blood-flecked sputum. A chest x-ray shows an opaque left upper lobe. He had several respiratory infections in his first year requiring admission to hospital.

On examination, there are decreased breath sounds in the left upper lobe and there are widespread crepitations throughout the left lung.

After treatment with antibiotics his fever resolves but his chest x-ray shows a hyperlucent left lung. A lung scan is performed, which shows markedly decreased perfusion of the left lung, but with normal ventilation.

Questions

1 What is the diagnosis?
2 What is the differential diagnosis?
3 What investigations are indicated?

Answers to case sixty-six

1 *Charcot–Marie–Tooth disease (peroneal muscular atrophy). Typically, he has gradual onset of gait abnormality, foot drop, dyspnoea, distal muscle wasting, absent reflexes and a classic distribution of sensory loss. His neonatal history and his CSF findings are non-contributory.*
Also consider diastematomyelia.

2 *a Nerve conduction (slowed).*
b cerebral CAT scan.
c Myelography.
d Spinal x-rays.

3 *The pattern of inheritance is variable and is not clear in this case.*

A 17-month-old Caucasian girl is admitted for investigation of poor appetite and poor weight gain. In recent weeks, she had become increasingly sleepy and irritable. There had been no diarrhoea or vomiting and no apparent difficulty with swallowing.

Past medical history: born after a full term normal delivery. Birth weight 2.2 kg. There were no neonatal problems. Bottle fed from birth, taking 'humanized' milk. She had fed well and gained weight normally until 7 months. Solid food had been introduced at 4 months. There were no other illnesses and her development was normal.

Development: sat at 9 months, walked at 13 months.

Family history: mother 21, well; father 22, a canteen assistant. The parents are separated and the child lives with her own mother. There is a sister, aged 5, who is well.

On examination, she was small and thin. Weight less than the 1st centile. She is noisy, uncooperative and difficult to examine. Neurologically she is normal and there are no other abnormalities.

Investigations

Haemoglobin	10 g/dl
MVC	81 fl
MCHC	34%
Serum folate	2 ng/ml
Urine culture negative	
Bone age	6 months
Serum iron	5.5 μmol/l
TIBC	60 μmol/l
Saturation	9.1%
Albumin	40 g/l

Questions

1 What is the differential diagnosis?
2 What further investigations would you suggest?
3 What comment would you make if she gained weight in hospital?

Answers to case sixty-seven

1 Diabetes inspidus. The onset is recent and her neonatal problems are unrelated.

2 Hand–Schüller–Christian disease.
Suggestive features are:

a her diabetes insipidus.
b proptosis.
c absence of evidence of raised intracranial pressure.
d normal BP.
e hepatomegaly.

Also consider a brain tumour, either primary or secondary, neuroblastoma or leukaemia.

3 a Vasopressin analogue (e.g. DDAVP) stimulation test.
b Early morning osmolality.
c Skull x-rays.
d Bone marrow aspiration.
e Cerebral CAT scan.
f Chest x-ray.

A 5-year-old Caucasian boy is admitted following a 10-day history of generalized urticaria which is diagnosed as insect bites by the general practitioner. He is brought to hospital following an episode of abdominal pain, with subsequent passage of several bloody, mucoid stools.

He has had several previous admissions with abdominal pain and his appendix was removed during one of these admissions. It was not inflamed. He gets travel sickness, but is otherwise healthy. Mother has migraine and father had asthma as a child. There are no siblings; however, there is a canary in the house.

On examination, he is febrile and unwell. There is an urticarial rash on the limbs and his abdomen is tender, maximally in the right iliac fossa. There are no limb or joint abnormalities and no loin tenderness. He is neurologically normal. His throat is slightly inflamed, but there are no cervical nodes palpable.

Questions

1 What is the diagnosis?
2 What three investigations would you suggest?
3 Is long term follow-up necessary?

Answers to case sixty-eight

1 *McLeod's syndrome. Features to suggest this diagnosis are his recurrent chest infections as an infant, his bloody sputum, presence of crepitations and his abnormal lung scan.*

2 a *Bronchiectasis.*
  b *Foreign body.*
  c *Hypogammaglobulinaemia.*
  d *Tuberculosis.*
  e *Cystic fibrosis.*
  f *Kartagener's syndrome.*
  g *Asthma.*
  h *Recurrent aspiration syndrome.*

3 a *Bronchoscopy.*
  b *Gastric washings for acid fast bacilli.*
  c *X-ray sinuses.*
  d *Pulmonary function.*
  e *Sweat test.*
  f *Serum immunoglobulins.*
  g *Barium swallow.*
  h *Ciliary biopsy.*
  i *Mantoux test.*

A 6-month-old Indian baby presents with a 4-day history of constipation. She had vomited on the day of admission and since then had been given nothing but water. On further questioning, her parents revealed that she had been coughing persistently since birth, and recently she had become tired while feeding.

She was born at 40 weeks' gestation, and was bottle fed from birth. Neonatal jaundice was treated with phototherapy and resolved completely. Both parents are well and there are no siblings. No family history of note.

On examination, she was tachypnoeic, 50 breaths/min, with slight intercostal recession. There was a soft systolic ejection murmur at the left sternal edge but normal peripheral pulses. There was palpable stool in the descending colon and slight hepatomegaly. She was floppy, had absent tendon reflexes and was unable to sit even with help.

She was treated with laxatives and had a normal bowel action. Over the next 2 days she became gradually more tachypnoeic, developing a gallop rhythm and further hepatomegaly.

Questions

1 What is the most likely diagnosis?
2 What investigations would you find most helpful?
3 How would you treat her?

Answers to case sixty-nine

1 *Many chronic disorders need consideration but the following in particular require exclusion:*
   a *Coeliac disease.*
   b *Poor dietary intake.*
   c *Cystic fibrosis.*
   d *Renal failure.*
   e *Hypothyroidism.*

(Think FTT DD)

2 a *Observation in hospital.*
   b *Jejunal biopsy.*
   c *Chest x-ray.*
   d *Immunoglobulins.*
   e *Serum T_4, TSH.*
   f *Electrolytes, creatinine.*
   g *Sweat electrolytes.*
   h *Differential sugar absorption.*

3 *Suspect nutritional and emotional deprivation as a cause particularly if weight gain in hospital exceeds the normal (i.e. 50 g/day at this age).*

A boy is born at 37 weeks' gestation by Caesarean section for pre-eclampsia, birth weight 2.8 kg, placental weight 1.2 kg. Apart from requiring brief intubation at delivery, he progresses normally, feeds well with good weight gain and he is discharged after 8 days. Mother continues breast feeding at home. He is apparently well until aged 6 weeks, when he presents with recurrent focal fits, which are brief and do not seem to distress him. He is asymptomatic between these episodes.

Both parents, from Turkey, are unrelated and are well. Two siblings, girls of 15 and 16, also well. A boy died at 6 weeks of age of unknown cause.

On examination, focal fits are observed, although he is otherwise neurologically normal. There is a pansystolic murmur at the apex and slight abdominal distension with ascites. The liver is palpable 2 cm below the right costal margin and the spleen is also just palpable.

While in hospital, his ascites becomes rather more marked but his fits, which are treated with calcium supplements, resolve.

Investigations

Calcium	1.4 mmol/l
Magnesium	0.36 mmol/l
Sugar	5.0 mmol/l
Haemoglobin	10.2 g/dl
Sodium	125 mmol/l

CSF examination – 1 white cell/mm^3, protein 0.15 g/l, sugar 2.8 mmol/l.

Questions

1 What is the underlying disease?
2 What is the prognosis?
3 What three tests would confirm the diagnosis?

Answers to case seventy

1 Intussusception associated with Henoch–Schönlein purpura.

2 a Barium enema.
b Full blood count and platelet count.
c Blood culture.

3 These patients may develop glomerulonephritis which may not present for several years. Depression may be a sequela. The intussusception is unlikely to recur.

A 1-month-old baby born to newly arrived Pakistani immigrants presents with fits during the week prior to admission. Breast fed, the baby is well and feeds adequately between fits, which occur about 10 times per day.

He was born at 36 weeks' gestation after a breech delivery, birth weight 2.8 kg. The baby required intubation initially, but responded well and was breathing spontaneously at 10 minutes. Apgar scores were 2 at 1 minute, 7 at 5 minutes. He was jaundiced at 2 days, requiring phototherapy but was discharged at 8 days, feeding well.

On examination, he is well with no physical abnormalities. The fontanelle is normotensive, there is no bruising or haematomata. He is observed to have several multifocal fits during the examination.

Questions

1 What is the most likely cause for the fits?
2 What investigations are required?
3 What treatment would you institute?

Answers to case seventy-one

1 This baby has cardiac failure complicating Pompe's disease. Features suggesting this underlying process are the deterioration after a normal neonatal period, her present hypotonicity, hepatomegaly and the development of cardiac failure.
Other possible diagnoses include:

a myocarditis and myositis (coxsackie virus).
b endocardial fibroelastosis.
c hypertrophic obstructive cardiomyopathy.

These are less likely because of her abnormal neurological examination.

2 a ECG (shows short P–R interval and left or combined venticular hypertrophy).
b Echocardiogram.
c Viral studies and serology.
d Fibroblast culture for enzyme assay (alpha-1,4-glucosidase).
e Cardiac catheterization.

3 a Acute failure:

i frusemide,
ii nasogastric feeding,
iii O$_2$,
iv perhaps ventilatory support,
v digoxin may be helpful.

b The long term prognosis is poor, most dying by 2 years. Treat each episode of failure and chest infections aggressively. The family will need continued support.

A 5-year-old Caucasian boy is seen for review in the outpatient clinic. Previously referred because of poor appetite and lack of energy, he was found to have mild motor retardation and hepatomegaly. Subsequently his symptoms resolved completely and his development has been normal. He is now doing well at school. There have been no episodes of drowsiness, loss of consciousness or fits. His hepatomegaly, however, is still present but less marked. Both parents are well and unrelated. A brother also has a large liver.

Questions

1 What is the likely diagnosis?
2 What investigations are necessary to confirm this?
3 What would you expect an ECG to show?

**Answers to
case seventy-two**

1 *This baby has the congenital nephrotic syndrome. The ascites, and the high placental weight, often 40% of the baby's weight, are typical features. The low calcium is common, although the ionized calcium is usually normal. Here, the hypocalcaemic fits are atypical.*

The commonest cause is the autosomal recessive Finnish type, but also consider congenital infection, e.g. syphilis and hepatitis B. A rare diffuse mesangial sclerosis has also been described.

2 *Almost invariably fatal. The response to corticosteroids and cyclophosphamide is poor. A raised alphafetoprotein in amniotic fluid allows antenatal diagnosis.*

3 a *Urinary and serum proteins.*
   b *Renal biopsy.*
   c *Serological tests for congenital infection.*
   d *Check thyroid status since these children are prone to hypothyroidism through excessive thyroid binding globulin loss.*

A 5-year-old girl was admitted with a 4-week history of limp and pain in the right foot. X-ray of the foot and ankle was normal; however, the foot remained painful and swollen and 2 weeks later an inguinal lymphadenopathy developed. She also developed nocturnal fever with sweats.

Investigations at that time

Haemoglobin	9.0 g/dl
White cell count	5×10^9/l
ESR	45 mm/h
GFR	76 ml/min

There was no proteinuria.

A diagnosis was made and she was treated appropriately. However, she was readmitted at 10 years of age with a 2-week history of malaise, fever and facial rash. On examination, she was found to be in cardiac failure with cardiomegaly, a gallop rhythm and bilateral pleural effusions. An ECG showed inverted T waves with ST elevation.

Past medical history: full term, normal delivery, birth weight 3.5 kg. No neonatal problem and no other serious illnesses.

The parents are well. They both are from the West Indies. There is one sibling, a girl of 14, also well.

Questions

1 What is the likely diagnosis?
2 What other diagnostic possibilities are there?
3 What three further investigations would you suggest to confirm the diagnosis?

Answers to case seventy-three

1 This baby has hypocalcaemia secondary to maternal hypocalcaemia. The syndrome is common in the immigrant population where there is poor maternal nutrition and the baby is fully breast fed. The absence of other neurological signs helps exclude an underlying neurological pathology.

2 a Total serum calcium and ionized calcium.
b Blood sugar.
c Serum magnesium.
d Blood count.
e Electrolytes and bicarbonate.
f Maternal vitamin D and calcium levels.
g Congenital infection antibody screen.
h Fundoscopy.

3 a Intravenous and oral calcium supplements.
b Vitamin D to mother and baby.
Most hypocalcaemic fits do not produce long term sequelae. However, 10% will have further, non-hypocalcaemic fits. The low 1 minute Apgar scores should not affect this baby's neurological status outside the immediate neonatal period.

A baby is born at term by spontaneous vaginal delivery, birth weight 3.8 kg. There has been no pre-existing fetal distress. Apgar scores are 2 at 1 minute, 3 at 5 minutes. He is intubated with difficulty and artificial ventilation is established at 10 minutes of age. He is given intravenous dextrose, bicarbonate and nalorphine, but his Apgar score is only 6 at 15 minutes.

At 1 hour of age, he still requires ventilatory support because of poor respiratory effort. He is pale with poor peripheral pulses and there is a loud pansystolic murmur over the praecordium.

At 8 hours there is spontaneous respiration, but he is hypotonic and is having repeated convulsions. These are treated with phenobarbitone.

At 16 hours there are poor pulses, poor cardiac output, hepatomegaly and he is treated with antibiotics and prostaglandins.

At 24 hours an ECG is performed, which is normal and a normal echocardiogram is also obtained. Plasma electrolyte results at this stage:

Sodium   120 mmol/l
Potassium   6.9 mmol/l
Urea   25.3 mmol/l

He is treated with tolazoline, dopamine, digoxin and frusemide with some improvement. He remains artificially ventilated, but stable haemodynamically. Nasojejunal feeds are introduced at 5 days.

At 9 days he is found to be more hypotonic, making no spontaneous movements. An infection screen, including lumbar puncture, is normal. A cerebral CAT scan is also normal.

At 15 days, he deteriorates suddenly and dies. A post mortem is performed.

Questions

1 What is found at post mortem?
2 What investigations should have been performed?
3 What is the correct treatment?

Answers to case seventy-four

1 A mild form of glycogenosis (III, VI or IX). This boy had Hers' disease (glycogenosis type VI; liver phosphorylase deficiency). It is unlikely to be type I, as the symptoms were mild, there was no hypoglycaemia and there was no stunting of growth. The regression of his hepatomegaly is typical.

2 a Leucocyte enzyme assay and red cell glycogen estimation.
*   b Liver biopsy – this normally shows vacuoles in the cytoplasm, glycogen staining with PAS, and low phosphorylase levels.*
*   c Usually normal fasting blood sugar level.*
*   d The glucose response to glucagon is normal or partially decreased.*
*   e Liver transaminase levels are normal or moderately elevated.*

3 Normal.

An 11-month-old Caucasian boy is brought to the casualty department with recurrent diarrhoea which has been present for the past 2 weeks. The stool contains flecks of bright blood, but no mucus and is very watery and yellow. He had initially been treated with a glucose/electrolyte mixture orally for 24 hours. Although the diarrhoea had resolved briefly, it had returned and persisted despite two further attempts to reintroduce normal feeds.

Past medical history: born at 36 weeks' gestation. Labour induced for Rhesus disease. An exchange transfusion had been performed and phototherapy given for 5 days. He had been bottle fed from birth. Solids were introduced at 4 months and doorstep milk at 7 months. There had been normal weight gain until this admission.

Family history: mother well, a midwife. Father has diabetes. Two siblings, boys of 3 and 6, both well.

On examination, he looks slightly wasted, but not dehydrated. His chest is clear. There is a small palpable spleen but no other masses, and the abdomen is soft.

Questions

1 What is the likely diagnosis?
2 What is the aetiology of the diarrhoea?
3 What is the correct management?

Answers to case seventy-five

1 Systemic lupus erythematosus (SLE), complicated by pericarditis.

2 a Tuberculosis.
  b Still's disease.
  c Rheumatic fever.
  d Sarcoidosis.

3 a LE cells.
  b Autoantibodies: ANF, RhF, anti-DNA.
  c Complement: C_3, C_4, CH50.
  d Mantoux.
  e Urine and gastric washings for acid fast bacilli.
  f Renal biopsy.
  g ECG
  h Echocardiogram.

A 14-year-old boy presents with several months of intermittent early morning weakness, usually occurring after the sports afternoon at school. He occasionally feels dyspnoeic during these episodes. After breakfast he is able to get dressed and go to school.

Past medical history: normal neonatal history – no hospital admissions. He has had mumps, measles and scarlet fever. He is doing well at school and there are no problems with vision or coordination and no history of headaches.

Family history: mother is a single parent who works as a teacher. There are no siblings. No family history known.

On examination, he appears well. He is of normal intelligence. Power, tone and reflexes are normal and his sensation is intact. He is observed in hospital and an attack of weakness occurs. During this episode, he is generally hypotonic and areflexic.

Questions

1 What is the diagnosis?
2 What investigations would you suggest?
3 What treatment is required?
4 What is the underlying pathophysiology?

Answers to case seventy-six

1 Bilateral adrenal haemorrhage secondary to neonatal asphyxia. The diagnosis can be difficult and needs to be distinguished from renal vein thrombosis, and in fact, it is unusual for even gross adrenal haemorrhage to cause an Addisonian state.

2 a Urinary cortisol.
b Serum 17-alpha-hydroxyprogesterone.
c Abdominal ultrasound will show enlarged adrenal glands, which may also be felt by palpation.
d IVP shows depression of the kidney on the affected side, with calyceal depression. Adrenal calcification may be present as early as the 5th day.

3 Immediate steroid replacement with cortisol hemisuccinate. Later, following saline replacement, hydrocortisone and perhaps 9-alpha-fludrocortisone.

A 4-year-old boy is referred to the casualty department following an episode of haematemesis. Two weeks previously he had been jaundiced with general malaise. The jaundice was resolving when he developed a cough and runny nose, for which his mother gave him a proprietary cough medicine. The following day his mother had noticed him to be pale and tired and not eating well. There had been dark stools and on the day of admission he had vomited half a cup of dark blood. He had been pale and listless since then, with abdominal pain.

He was bottle fed from birth and solids were introduced at three months. There were no other illnesses. He was born at 38 weeks' gestation, birth weight 3.1 kg.

Both parents are healthy and there is no family history of illness.

On examination, he is pale, but alert and cooperative. There are no petechiae or spider naevi and no jaundice. Heart rate 160 beats/min and blood pressure 100/60 mmHg. The abdomen is soft, the liver is palpable 2 cm below the right costal margin. There are no other masses.

Questions

1 What is the most likely cause of the initial episode and the underlying problem?
2 What is the differential diagnosis?
3 What five investigations would you suggest?
4 What is the appropriate treatment?

Answers to case seventy-seven

1 Post-enteritis enteropathy. The history is typical: an acute episode of infective diarrhoea with return of symptoms when a normal diet is reintroduced.

2 Initially an infection, either viral (rota, adeno, corona, or entero) or bacterial (E. coli, Shigella, Yersinia, Salmonella or Campylobacter). Subsequently it is due to lactose or cows' milk protein intolerance.

3 Test for sugar and pH in stools. Feed with a lactose-free, cows' milk formula. If symptoms persist, change to a soya-based lactose-free formula.
It is usual to attempt to confirm the diagnosis by rechallenge with cows' milk after weight gain has been consolidated.
A small bowel biopsy may be helpful.

A 6-month-old girl is admitted with acute onset of diarrhoea, flushing and loss of consciousness. She has had several previous mild episodes since 1 week of age, and all were associated with irritability and refusing feeds. There had been no fits.

Her neonatal history was uncomplicated following a full term normal delivery, birth weight 3.2 kg.

Two maternal cousins died with neutropenia, but the immediate family is well and their own immunological function is normal.

On examination, her height and weight are on the 25th centile. Blood pressure 100/60 mmHg and remains normal despite further episodes of flushing. There are no abdominal masses and she has three small raised macules on the left leg. In addition to a port wine stain on the right side of her face, she also has a mild strabismus.

Investigations

Full blood count normal
Immunoglobulins normal
Skeletal survey normal
Chest x-ray normal

Questions

1 What is the diagnosis?
2 What three tests would confirm this?
3 What treatment would you suggest?

Answers to case seventy-eight

1 Hypokalaemic familial periodic paralysis. This is suggested by the episodic nature of his weakness, with long periods of normality. It is often precipitated by large meals and periods of inactivity after exercise. It is unlikely to be hyperkalaemic familial paralysis as this occurs in younger children and paralysis is more localized, e.g. one limb.

2 Serum potassium after exercise. It is low during an attack (less than 3 mmol/l).

3 Potassium supplements.
Acetazolamide may also be effective.

4 Unknown. It is transmitted as an autosomal dominant, but is usually more severe in males. Attacks usually decrease with age.

Answers to case seventy-nine

1 This boy had suffered an acute gastric erosion following salicylate ingestion, preceded by infectious hepatitis. Remember that some proprietary cough medicines contain other non-antitussive additives; in this case, aspirin.

2 a Hepatitis proceeding to cirrhosis and oesophageal varices.
  b Leukaemia.
  c Infectious mononucleosis.

3 a Liver function tests.
  b Clotting studies.
  c Full blood count and platelet count.
  d Haptoglobins.
  e Reticulocyte count.
  f Chest x-ray.
  g Barium swallow and/or oesophagoscopy.
  h Heterophile antibodies (Paul Bunnell).

4 a Blood transfusion.
  b Fresh frozen plasma.
  c Cimetidine.
  d Antacids.
  e Vitamin K.

Warn the mother regarding aspirin-containing preparations.

Answers to
case eighty

1 *Mastocytosis (urticaria pigmentosa), a sporadic condition characterized by accumulation of mast cells in the dermis and sometimes infiltration of other organs. Her history is characteristic: episodes of acute histamine release producing diarrhoea, flushing and irritability. The macules on her leg are infiltrates of mast cells.*

Her normal blood pressure, normal blood count and otherwise normal physical examination are against her having a phaeochromocytoma or neuroblastoma, although these are possible, and the skin lesions are not typical of the carcinoid syndrome.

2 a *Urinary 5-hydroxytryptamine.*
b *Urinary VMA.*
c *Biopsy skin lesions.*

3 a *Remove lesions if these are causing symptoms.*
b *Antihistamines.*
c *Cimetidine.*
d *Avoidance of triggering factors, e.g. skin stimulation, and drugs, e.g. opiates, polymyxin B and acetylsalicylic acid.*